Domestic Investigations and Operations Guide

Federal Bureau of Investigation

Domestic Investigations and Operations Guide

Federal Bureau of Investigation (FBI)

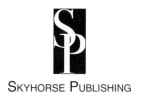

SKYHORSE PUBLISHING

First Skyhorse Publishing edition 2012.

Skyhorse Publishing books may be purchased in bulk at special discounts for sales promotion, corporate gifts, fund-raising, or educational purposes. Special editions can also be created to specifications. For details, contact the Special Sales Department, Skyhorse Publishing, 307 West 36th Street, 11th Floor, New York, NY 10018 or info@skyhorsepublishing.com.

Skyhorse® and Skyhorse Publishing® are registered trademarks of Skyhorse Publishing, Inc.®, a Delaware corporation.

Visit our website at www.skyhorsepublishing.com.

10 9 8 7 6 5 4 3 2 1

Library of Congress Cataloging-in-Publication Data is available on file.

Cover design by Adam Bozarth

Print ISBN: 978-1-63220-704-3
Ebook ISBN: 978-1-62636-605-3

Printed in China

Table of Contents

List of Appendices

(U) Preamble

December 1, 2008

(U) As the primary investigative agency of the federal government, the FBI has the authority and responsibility to investigate all violations of federal law that are not exclusively assigned to another federal agency. The FBI is further vested by law and by Presidential directives with the primary role in carrying out criminal investigations and investigations of threats to the national security of the United States. This includes the lead domestic role in investigating international terrorist threats to the United States, and in conducting counterintelligence activities to counter foreign entities' espionage and intelligence efforts directed against the United States. The FBI is also vested with important functions in collecting foreign intelligence as a member agency of the United States Intelligence Community (USIC). (AGG-Dom, Introduction)

(U) While investigating crime, terrorism, and threats to the national security, and collecting foreign intelligence, the FBI must fully comply with all laws and regulations, including those designed to protect civil liberties and privacy. Through compliance, the FBI will continue to earn the support, confidence and respect of the people of the United States.

(U) To assist the FBI in its mission, the Attorney General signed *The Attorney General's Guidelines for Domestic FBI Operations* (AGG-Dom) on September 29, 2008. The primary purpose of the AGG-Dom and the Domestic Investigations and Operations Guide (DIOG) is to standardize policy so that criminal, national security, and foreign intelligence investigative activities are accomplished in a consistent manner, whenever possible (e.g., same approval, notification, and reporting requirements). In addition to the DIOG, each FBIHQ substantive Division has a policy implementation guide (PG) that supplements this document. Numerous FBI manuals, electronic communications, letterhead memoranda, and other policy documents are incorporated into the DIOG and the substantive Division policy implementation guides, thus, consolidating the FBI's policy guidance. The FBIHQ Corporate Policy Office (CPO) plays an instrumental role in this endeavor. Specifically, the CPO maintains the most current version of the DIOG on its website. As federal statutes, executive orders, Attorney General guidelines, FBI policies, or other relevant authorities change, CPO will electronically update the DIOG after appropriate coordination and required approvals.

(U) The changes implemented by the DIOG should better equip you to protect the people of the United States against crime and threats to the national security and to collect foreign intelligence. This is your document, and it requires your input so that we can provide the best service to our nation. If you discover a need for change, please forward your suggestion to FBIHQ CPO.

(U) Thank you for your outstanding service!

Robert S. Mueller, III

Director

1. (U) Scope and Purpose

1.1. (U) Scope

(U) The DIOG applies to all investigative activities and intelligence collection activities conducted by the FBI within the United States or outside the territories of all countries. This policy document does not apply to investigative and intelligence collection activities of the FBI in foreign countries; those are governed by *The Attorney General's Guidelines for Extraterritorial FBI Operations.*

1.2. (U) Purpose

(U) The purpose of the DIOG is to standardize policy so that criminal, national security, and foreign intelligence investigative activities are consistently and uniformly accomplished whenever possible (e.g., same approval, notification, and reporting requirements).

(U) This policy document also stresses the importance of oversight and self-regulation to ensure that all investigative and intelligence collection activities are conducted within Constitutional and statutory parameters and that civil liberties and privacy are protected.

(U) In addition to this policy document, each FBIHQ substantive Division has a PG that supplements the DIOG. As a result, numerous FBI manuals, electronic communications, letterhead memoranda, and other policy documents are incorporated into the DIOG and Division PGs, thus, consolidating FBI policy guidance.

2. (U) General Authorities and Principles

2.1.   (U) Scope of the Attorney General's Guidelines for Domestic FBI Operations

(U) The *Attorney General's Guidelines for Domestic FBI Operations* (AGG-Dom) apply to investigative and intelligence collection activities conducted by the FBI within the United States, in the United States territories, or outside the territories of all countries. They do not apply to investigative and intelligence collection activities of the FBI in foreign countries, which will be governed by the *Attorney General's Guidelines for Extraterritorial FBI Operations*, when published. (Reference: AGG-Dom, Part I.A.)

(U) The AGG-Dom replaces the following six guidelines:

- *(U) The Attorney General's Guidelines on General Crimes, Racketeering Enterprise and Terrorism Enterprise Investigations* (May 30, 2002)

- *(U) The Attorney General's Guidelines for FBI National Security Investigations and Foreign Intelligence Collection* (October 31, 2003)

- *(U) The Attorney General's Supplemental Guidelines for Collection, Retention, and Dissemination of Foreign Intelligence* (November 29, 2006)

- *(U) The Attorney General Procedure for Reporting and Use of Information Concerning Violations of Law and Authorization for Participation in Otherwise Illegal Activity in FBI Foreign Intelligence, Counterintelligence or International Terrorism Intelligence Investigations* (August 8, 1988).

- *(U) The Attorney General's Guidelines for Reporting on Civil Disorders and Demonstrations Involving a Federal Interest* (April 5, 1976)

- *(U) The Attorney General's Procedures for Lawful, Warrantless Monitoring of Verbal Communications* (May 30, 2002) [only portion applicable to FBI repealed]

(U) The Attorney General will be issuing a separate set of new guidelines for extraterritorial operations, the *Attorney General's Guidelines for Extraterritorial FBI Operations*. However, certain of the existing guidelines that are repealed by the AGG-Dom currently apply in part to extraterritorial operations, including the *Attorney General's Guidelines for FBI National Security Investigations and Foreign Intelligence Collection*, and the *Attorney General Procedure for Reporting and Use of Information Concerning Violations of Law and Authorization for Participation in Otherwise Illegal Activity in FBI Foreign Intelligence, Counterintelligence or International Terrorism Intelligence Investigations*. To ensure that there is no gap in the existence of guidelines for extraterritorial operations, these existing guidelines will remain in effect in their application to extraterritorial operations until the *Attorney General's Guidelines for Extraterritorial FBI Operations* are issued and take effect, notwithstanding the general repeal of these existing guidelines by the AGG-Dom.

(U) Also, the classified *Attorney General Guidelines for Extraterritorial FBI Operation and Criminal Investigations* (1993) will continue to apply to FBI criminal investigations, pending the execution of the new guidelines for extraterritorial operations, as discussed above. Finally, for national security and foreign intelligence investigations, FBI investigative activities will continue to be processed as set forth in the classified *Memorandum of Understanding Concerning*

Overseas and Domestic Activities of the Central Intelligence Agency and the Federal Bureau of Investigation (2005).

2.2.   (U) General FBI Authorities under AGG-Dom

(U) The AGG-Dom recognizes four broad, general FBI authorities. (AGG-Dom, Part I.B.)

A. (U) Conduct Investigations and Collect Intelligence and Evidence

(U) The FBI is authorized to collect intelligence and to conduct investigations to detect, obtain information about, and prevent and protect against federal crimes and threats to the national security and to collect foreign intelligence, as provided in the DIOG (AGG-Dom, Part II).

(U) By regulation, the Attorney General has directed the FBI to investigate violations of the laws of the United States and collect evidence in cases in which the United States is or may be a party in interest, except in cases in which such responsibility is by statute or otherwise specifically assigned to another investigative agency. The FBI's authority to investigate and collect evidence involving criminal drug laws of the United States is concurrent with such authority of the Drug Enforcement Administration (28 C.F.R. § 0.85[a]).

B. (U) Provide Investigative Assistance

(U) The FBI is authorized to provide investigative assistance to other federal, state, local, or tribal agencies, and foreign agencies as provided in Section 12 of the DIOG (AGG-Dom, Part III).

C. (U) Conduct Strategic Analysis and Planning

(U) The FBI is authorized to conduct intelligence analysis and planning as provided in Section 15 of the DIOG (AGG-Dom, Part IV).

D. (U) Retain and Share Information

(U) The FBI is authorized to retain and share information obtained pursuant to the AGG-Dom, as provided in Section 14 of the DIOG (AGG-Dom, Part VI).

2.3.   (U) FBI as an Intelligence Agency

(U) The FBI is an intelligence agency as well as a law enforcement agency. Its basic functions accordingly extend beyond limited investigations of discrete matters, and include broader analytic and planning functions. The FBI's responsibilities in this area derive from various administrative and statutory sources. See Executive Order 12333; 28 U.S.C. § 532 note (incorporating P.L. 108-458 §§ 2001-2003) and 534 note (incorporating P.L. 109-162 § 1107).

(U) Part IV of the AGG-Dom authorizes the FBI to engage in intelligence analysis and planning, drawing on all lawful sources of information. The functions authorized under that Part includes: (i) development of overviews and analyses concerning threats to and vulnerabilities of the United States and its interests; (ii) research and analysis to produce reports and assessments (see note below) concerning matters relevant to investigative activities or other authorized FBI activities; and (iii) the operation of intelligence systems that facilitate and support investigations through the compilation and analysis of data and information on an ongoing basis.

(U) **Note:** In the DIOG, the word "assessment" has two distinct meanings. The AGG-Dom authorizes as an investigative activity an "assessment" which requires an authorized purpose as discussed in the DIOG Section 5. The United States Intelligence Community (USIC), however, also uses the word "assessment" to describe written intelligence products as discussed in the DIOG Section 15.7.B.

2.4. (U) FBI Lead Investigative Authorities

A. (U) Introduction

(U//FOUO) The FBI's primary investigative authority is derived from the authority of the Attorney General as provided in 28 U.S.C. §§ 509, 510, 533 and 534. Within this authority, the Attorney General may appoint officials to detect crimes against the United States and to conduct such other investigations regarding official matters under the control of the Department of Justice (DOJ) and the Department of State (DOS) as may be directed by the Attorney General (28 U.S.C. § 533). The Attorney General has delegated a number of his statutory authorities and granted other authorities to the Director of the FBI (28 C.F.R. § 0.85[a]). Some of these authorities apply both inside and outside the United States.

B. (U) Terrorism and Counterterrorism Investigations

(U) The Attorney General has directed the FBI to exercise Lead Agency responsibility in investigating all crimes for which DOJ has primary or concurrent jurisdiction and which involve terrorist activities or acts in preparation of terrorist activities within the statutory jurisdiction of the United States. Within the United States, this includes the collection, coordination, analysis, management and dissemination of intelligence and criminal information, as appropriate. If another federal agency identifies an individual who is engaged in terrorist activities or in acts in preparation of terrorist activities, the other agency is required to promptly notify the FBI. Terrorism, in this context, includes the unlawful use of force and violence against persons or property to intimidate or coerce a government, the civilian population, or any segment thereof, to further political or social objectives (28 C.F.R. § 0.85[a]).

C. (U) "Federal Crimes of Terrorism"

(U) Pursuant to the delegation in 28 C.F.R. § 0.85(a), the FBI exercises the Attorney General's lead investigative responsibility under 18 U.S.C. § 2332b(f) for all "federal crimes of terrorism" as identified in that statute. Many of these statutes grant the FBI extraterritorial investigative responsibility. Check the cited statute for the full particulars concerning elements of the offense, jurisdiction, etc. Under 18 U.S.C. § 2332b(g)(5), the term "federal crime of terrorism" means an offense that is: (i) calculated to influence or affect the conduct of government by intimidation or coercion or to retaliate against government conduct; and (ii) is a violation of federal statute relating to:

1. (U) Destruction of aircraft or aircraft facilities (18 U.S.C. § 32);

2. (U) Violence at international airports (applies to offenses occurring outside the United States in certain situations) (18 U.S.C. § 37);

3. (U) Arson within "special maritime and territorial jurisdiction of the United States" (SMTJ is defined in 18 U.S.C. § 7) (18 U.S.C. § 81);

4. (U) Prohibitions with respect to biological weapons (extraterritorial federal jurisdiction if offense committed by or against a United States national) (18 U.S.C. § 175);

5. (U) Possession of biological agents or toxins by restricted persons (18 U.S.C. § 175b);

6. (U) Variola virus (includes smallpox and other derivatives of the variola major virus) (applies to offenses occurring outside the United States in certain situations) (18 U.S.C. § 175c);

7. (U) Prohibited activities regarding chemical weapons (applies to offenses occurring outside the United States in certain situations) (18 U.S.C. § 229) (E.O. 13128 directs any possible violation of this statute be referred to the FBI);

8. (U) Congressional, Cabinet, and Supreme Court assassination, kidnapping and assault (18 U.S.C. § 351[a]-[d]) (18 U.S.C. § 351[g] directs that the FBI shall investigate violations of this statute);

9. (U) Prohibited transactions involving nuclear materials (applies to offenses occurring outside the United States in certain situations) (18 U.S.C. § 831);

10. (U) Participation in nuclear and weapons of mass destruction threats to the United States (extraterritorial federal jurisdiction) (18 U.S.C. § 832);

11. (U) Importation, exportation, shipping, transport, transfer, receipt, or possession of plastic explosives that do not contain a detection agent (18 U.S.C. § 842[m] and [n]);

12. (U) Arson or bombing of government property risking or causing death (18 U.S.C. § 844[f][2] or [3]) (18 U.S.C. § 846[a] grants FBI and the Bureau of Alcohol, Tobacco, Firearms, and Explosives (ATF) concurrent authority to investigate violations of this statute);

13. (U) Arson or bombing of property used in or affecting interstate or foreign commerce (18 U.S.C. § 844[i]) (18 U.S.C. § 846[a] grants FBI and ATF concurrent authority to investigate violations of this statute);

14. (U) Killing or attempted killing during an attack on a federal facility with a dangerous weapon (18 U.S.C. § 930[c]);

15. (U) Conspiracy within United States jurisdiction to murder, kidnap, or maim persons at any place outside the United States (18 U.S.C. § 956[a][1]);

16. (U) Using a computer for unauthorized access, transmission, or retention of protected information (18 U.S.C. § 1030[a][1]) (18 U.S.C. § 1030[d][2] grants the FBI "primary authority" to investigate Section 1030[a][1] offenses involving espionage, foreign counterintelligence, information protected against unauthorized disclosure for reasons of national defense or foreign relations, or Restricted Data as defined in the Atomic Energy Act, except for offenses affecting United States Secret Service (USSS) duties under 18 U.S.C. § 3056[a]);

17. (U) Knowingly transmitting a program, information, code, or command and thereby intentionally causing damage, without authorization, to a protected computer (18 U.S.C. § 1030[a][5][A][i]);

18. (U) Killing or attempted killing of officers or employees of the United States, including any member of the uniformed services (18 U.S.C. § 1114);

19. (U) Murder or manslaughter of foreign officials, official guests, or international, protected persons (applies to offenses occurring outside the United States in certain situations) (18 U.S.C. § 1116) (Attorney General may request military assistance in the course of enforcement of this section);

20. (U) Hostage taking (applies to offenses occurring outside the United States in certain situations) (18 U.S.C. § 1203);

21. (U) Willfully injuring or committing any depredation against government property or contracts (18 U.S.C. § 1361);

22. (U) Destruction of communication lines, stations, or systems (18 U.S.C. § 1362);

23. (U) Destruction or injury to buildings or property within special maritime and territorial jurisdiction of the United States (18 U.S.C. § 1363);

24. (U) Destruction of $100,000 or more of an "energy facility" property as defined in the statute (18 U.S.C. § 1366);

25. (U) Presidential and Presidential staff assassination, kidnapping, and assault (18 U.S.C. § 1751[a], [b], [c], or [d]) (extraterritorial jurisdiction) (Per 18 U.S.C. § 1751[i], 1751 violations must be investigated by the FBI; FBI may request assistance from any federal [including military], state, or local agency notwithstanding any statute, rule, or regulation to the contrary);

26. (U) Terrorist attacks and other violence against railroad carriers and against mass transportation systems on land, on water, or through the air (includes a school bus, charter, or sightseeing transportation; or any means of transport on land, water, or through the air) (18 U.S.C. § 1992);

27. (U) Destruction of national defense materials, premises, or utilities (18 U.S.C. § 2155);

28. (U) Production of defective national defense materials, premises, or utilities (18 U.S.C. § 2156);

29. (U) Violence against maritime navigation (18 U.S.C. § 2280);

30. (U) Violence against maritime fixed platforms (located on the continental shelf of the United States or located internationally in certain situations) (18 U.S.C. § 2281);

31. (U) Certain homicides and other violence against United States nationals occurring outside of the United States (18 U.S.C. § 2332);

32. (U) Use of weapons of mass destruction (against a national of the United States while outside the United States; against certain persons or property within the United States; or by a national of the United States outside the United States) (18 U.S.C. § 2332a) (WMD defined in 18 U.S.C. § 2332a[c][2]);

33. (U) Acts of terrorism transcending national boundaries (includes murder, kidnapping, and other prohibited acts occurring inside and outside the United States under specified circumstances – including that the victim is a member of a uniform service; includes offenses committed in the United States territorial sea and airspace above and seabed below; includes offenses committed in special maritime and territorial jurisdiction of the United States as defined in 18 U.S.C. § 7) (18 U.S.C. § 2332b);

34. (U) Bombings of places of public use, government facilities, public transportation systems and infrastructure facilities (applies to offenses occurring inside or outside the United States in certain situations; does not apply to activities of armed forces during an armed conflict) (18 U.S.C. § 2332f);

35. (U) Missile systems designed to destroy aircraft (applies to offenses occurring outside the United States in certain situations) (18 U.S.C. § 2332g);

36. (U) Radiological dispersal devices (applies to offenses occurring outside the United States in certain situations) (18 U.S.C. § 2332h);

37. (U) Harboring or concealing terrorists (18 U.S.C. § 2339);

38. (U) Providing material support or resources to terrorists (18 U.S.C. § 2339A);

39. (U) Providing material support or resources to designated foreign terrorist organizations (extraterritorial federal jurisdiction) (18 U.S.C. § 2339B) ("The Attorney General shall conduct any investigation of a possible violation of this section, or of any license, order, or regulation issued pursuant to this section." 18 U.S.C. § 2339B[e][1]);

40. (U) Prohibitions against the financing of terrorism (applies to offenses occurring outside the United States in certain situations including on board a vessel flying the flag of the United States or an aircraft registered under the laws of the United States) (18 U.S.C. § 2339C) (Memorandum of Agreement between the Attorney General and the Secretary of Homeland Security, dated May 13, 2005: FBI leads all terrorist financing investigations and operations);

41. (U) Relating to military-type training from a foreign terrorist organization (extraterritorial jurisdiction) (18 U.S.C. § 2339D);

42. (U) Torture applies only to torture committed outside the United States in certain situations; torture is defined in 18 U.S.C. § 2340 (18 U.S.C. § 2340A);

43. (U) Prohibitions governing atomic weapons (applies to offenses occurring outside the United States in certain situations) (42 U.S.C. § 2122) (FBI shall investigate alleged or suspected violations per 42 U.S.C. § 2271[b]);

44. (U) Sabotage of nuclear facilities or fuel (42 U.S.C. § 2284) (FBI shall investigate alleged or suspected violations per 42 U.S.C. § 2271[b]);

45. (U) Aircraft piracy (applies to offenses occurring outside the United States in certain situations) (49 U.S.C. § 46502) (FBI shall investigate per 28 U.S.C. § 538);

46. (U) Assault on a flight crew with a dangerous weapon (applies to offenses occurring in the "special aircraft jurisdiction of the United States" as defined in 49 U.S.C. § 46501[2]); (second sentence of 49 U.S.C. § 46504) (FBI shall investigate per 28 U.S.C. § 538);

47. (U) Placement of an explosive or incendiary device on an aircraft (49 U.S.C. § 46505[b][3]) (FBI shall investigate per 28 U.S.C. § 538);

48. (U) Endangerment of human life on aircraft by means of weapons (49 U.S.C. § 46505[c]) (FBI shall investigate per 28 U.S.C. § 538);

49. (U) Application of certain criminal laws to acts on aircraft (if homicide or attempted homicide is involved) (applies to offenses occurring in the "special aircraft jurisdiction of

the United States" as defined in 18 U.S.C. § 46501[2]); (49 U.S.C. § 46506) (FBI shall investigate per 28 U.S.C. § 538);

50. (U) Damage or destruction of interstate gas or hazardous liquid pipeline facility (49 U.S.C. § 60123[b]); and

51. (U) Section 1010A of the Controlled Substances Import and Export Act (relating to narco-terrorism).

D. (U) **Additional offenses not defined as "Federal Crimes of Terrorism"**

(U) Title 18 U.S.C. § 2332b(f) expressly grants the Attorney General primary investigative authority for additional offenses not defined as "Federal Crimes of Terrorism." These offenses are (**Note:** nothing in this section of the DIOG may be construed to interfere with the USSS under 18 U.S.C. § 3056):

1. (U) Congressional, Cabinet, and Supreme Court assaults (18 U.S.C. § 351[e]) (18 U.S.C. § 351[g]) directs that the FBI investigate violations of this statute);

2. (U) Using mail, telephone, telegraph, or other instrument of interstate or foreign commerce to threaten to kill, injure, or intimidate any individual, or unlawfully to damage or destroy any building, vehicle, or other real or personal property by means of fire or explosive (18 U.S.C. § 844[e]); (18 U.S.C. § 846[a] grants FBI and ATF concurrent authority to investigate violations of this statute);

3. (U) Damages or destroys by means of fire or explosive any building, vehicle, or other personal or real property, possessed, owned, or leased to the United States or any agency thereof, or any institution receiving federal financial assistance (18 U.S.C. § 844[f][1]) (18 U.S.C. § 846[a] grants FBI and ATF concurrent authority to investigate violations of this statute);

4. (U) Conspiracy within United States jurisdiction to damage or destroy property in a foreign country and belonging to a foreign country, or to any railroad, canal, bridge, airport, airfield, or other public utility, public conveyance, or public structure, or any religious, educational, or cultural property so situated (18 U.S.C. § 956[b]);

5. (U) Destruction of $5,000 or more of an "energy facility" property as defined in 18 U.S.C. § 1366(c) (18 U.S.C. § 1366[b]); and

6. (U) Willful trespass upon, injury to, destruction of, or interference with fortifications, harbor defenses, or defensive sea areas (18 U.S.C. § 2152).

E. (U//FOUO) **NSPD-46/HSPD-15, "U.S. Policy and Strategy in the War on Terror"**

(U//FOUO) Annex II (Consolidation and Updating of Outdated Presidential Counterterrorism Documents), dated January 10, 2007, to National Security Presidential Directive (NSPD) 46/Homeland Security Presidential Directive (HSPD) 15, dated March 6, 2006, establishes FBI lead responsibilities, as well as those of other federal entities, in the "War on Terror."

(U//FOUO) Areas addressed in Annex II[   ]   b2
[   ]   b7E
[   ] Both NSPD-
46/HSPD-15 and Annex II thereto are classified.

(U) Counterintelligence and Espionage Investigations

(U//FOUO) A representative list of federal statutes applicable to counterintelligence and espionage investigations appears below. For additional information, refer to the Counterintelligence Program Implementation Guide and the current list of espionage and counterintelligence authorities.

1. (U) **Espionage Investigations of Persons in United States Diplomatic Missions Abroad**

   (U) Section 603 of the Intelligence Authorization Act of 1990 (P.L. 101-193) states that, subject to the authority of the Attorney General, "the FBI shall supervise the conduct of all investigations of violations of the espionage laws of the United States by persons employed by or assigned to United States diplomatic missions abroad. All departments and agencies shall provide appropriate assistance to the FBI in the conduct of such investigations." Consult the Attorney General's extraterritorial guidelines and other applicable policy or agreements.

2. (U) **Investigations of Unauthorized Disclosure of Classified Information to a Foreign Power or Agent of a Foreign Power**

   (U) The National Security Act of 1947, as amended, establishes procedures for the coordination of counterintelligence activities (50 U.S.C. § 402a). Part of that statute requires that, absent extraordinary circumstances as approved by the President in writing on a case-by-case basis, the head of each executive branch department or agency must ensure that the FBI is "advised immediately of any information, regardless of its origin, which indicates that classified information is being, or may have been, disclosed in an unauthorized manner to a foreign power or an agent of a foreign power."

G. (U) Criminal Investigations

(U//FOUO) In addition to the statutes listed above and below, refer to the Criminal Investigative Division (CID) Program Implementation Guide (PG) for additional criminal jurisdiction information.

1. (U) **Investigations of aircraft privacy and related violations**

   (U) The FBI shall investigate any violation of 49 U.S.C. § 46314 (Entering aircraft or airport areas in violation of security requirements) or chapter 465 (Special aircraft jurisdiction of the United States) of Title 49, United States Code. (28 U.S.C. § 538)

2. (U) **Violent crimes against foreign travelers**

   (U) The Attorney General and Director of the FBI shall assist state and local authorities in investigating and prosecuting a felony crime of violence in violation of the law of any State in which the victim appears to have been selected because he or she is a traveler from a foreign nation. (28 U.S.C. § 540A[b])

3. (U) Felonious killings of state and local law enforcement officers (28 U.S.C. § 540); and

4. (U) Investigations of serial killings (28 U.S.C. § 540I

H. (U) Authority of an FBI Special Agent

(U) An FBI Special Agent has the authority to:

1. (U) Investigate violations of the laws, including the criminal drug laws, of the United States (21 U.S.C. § 871; 28 U.S.C. §§ 533, 534 and 535; 28 C.F.R. § 0.85).

2. (U) Collect evidence in cases in which the United States is or may be a party in interest (28 C.F.R. § 0.85 [a]) as redelegated through exercise of the authority contained in 28 C.F.R. § 0.138 to direct personnel in the FBI.

3. (U) Make arrests (18 U.S.C. §§ 3052 and 3062).

4. (U) Serve and execute arrest warrants and seize property under warrant; issue and/or serve administrative subpoenas; serve subpoenas issued by other proper authority; and make civil investigative demands (18 U.S.C. §§ 3052, 3107; 21 U.S.C. § 876; 15 U.S.C. § 1312).

5. (U) Carry firearms (18 U.S.C. § 3052).

6. (U) Administer oaths to witnesses attending to testify or depose in the course of investigations of frauds on or attempts to defraud the United States or irregularities or misconduct of employees or agents of the United States (5 U.S.C. § 303).

7. (U) Seize property subject to seizure under the criminal and civil forfeiture laws of the United States (e.g., 18 U.S.C. §§ 981 and 982).

8. (U) Perform other duties imposed by law.

2.5. (U) Status as Internal Guidance

(U) The AGG-Dom and this DIOG are set forth solely for the purpose of internal DOJ and FBI guidance. They are not intended to, do not, and may not be relied upon to create any rights, substantive or procedural, enforceable by law by any party in any matter, civil or criminal, nor do they place any limitation on otherwise lawful investigative and litigative prerogatives of the DOJ and the FBI. (AGG-Dom, Part I.D.2.)

2.6. (U) Departures from the AGG-Dom

A. (U//FOUO) **Departure from the AGG-Dom in Advance of an Operation:** A Departure from the AGG-Dom must be approved by the Director of the FBI, by the Deputy Director of the FBI, or by an Executive Assistant Director (EAD) designated by the Director. The Director of the FBI has designated the EAD National Security Branch or the EAD Criminal Cyber Response and Services Branch to grant departures from the AGG-Dom. Notice of the departure must be provided to the General Counsel (GC).

B. (U//FOUO) **Emergency Exception for a Departure from the AGG-Dom:** If a departure from the AGG-Dom is necessary without such prior approval because of the immediacy or gravity of a threat to the safety of persons or property or to the national security, the Director, the Deputy Director, or a designated EAD, and the GC must be notified by the official granting the emergency departure as soon thereafter as practicable. The FBI must provide timely written notice of departures from the AGG-Dom to the DOJ Criminal Division or

National Security Division (NSD), as appropriate, and the Criminal Division or NSD must notify the Attorney General and the Deputy Attorney General. Notwithstanding this paragraph, all activities in all circumstances must be carried out in a manner consistent with the Constitution and laws of the United States. (AGG-Dom, Part I.D.3.)

C. (U//FOUO) **Records of Departures from the AGG-Dom:** The Office of the General Counsel (OGC) is responsible for maintaining records of all requests and approvals or denials of departures from the AGG-Dom.

2.7. (U) Departures from the DIOG

A. (U//FOUO) **Departure from the DIOG in Advance of an Operation:** A request for a "departure from" any provision of the DIOG must be submitted to the appropriate substantive program Assistant Director (AD) and to the GC for approval prior to exercising a departure from the DIOG. The AD may designate the Deputy Assistant Director (DAD), and the GC may designate the Deputy General Counsel for the National Security Law Branch (NSLB) or the Deputy General Counsel for the Investigative Law Branch (ILB) to approve departures. Notwithstanding this paragraph, all activities in all circumstances must be carried out in a manner consistent with the Constitution and laws of the United States.

B. (U//FOUO) **Emergency Exception for a Departure from the DIOG:** If a departure is necessary because of the immediacy or gravity of a threat to the safety of persons or property or to the national security, the approving authority may, at his/her discretion, authorize an emergency departure from the DIOG. As soon as practicable thereafter, the Special Agent in Charge (SAC) or FBIHQ Section Chief must provide, in writing, notice to the appropriate AD and GC describing the circumstances and necessity for the departure. Notwithstanding this paragraph, all activities in all circumstances must be carried out in a manner consistent with the Constitution and laws of the United States.

C. (U//FOUO) **Records of Departures from the DIOG:** The OGC is responsible for maintaining records of all requests and approvals or denials of departures from the DIOG.

2.8. (U) Other FBI Activities Not Limited by AGG-Dom

(U) The AGG-Dom apply to FBI investigative activities as provided herein and do not limit other authorized activities of the FBI, such as the FBI's responsibilities to conduct background checks and inquiries concerning applicants and employees under federal personnel security programs (e.g., background investigations), the FBI's maintenance and operation of national criminal records systems and preparation of national crime statistics, and the forensic assistance and administration functions of the FBI Laboratory. (AGG-Dom, Part I.D.4.)

(U) FBI employees may incidentally obtain information relating to matters outside of the FBI's primary investigative responsibility. For example, information relating to violations of state or local law or foreign law may be incidentally obtained in the course of investigating federal crimes or threats to the national security or in collecting foreign intelligence. The AGG-Dom does not bar the acquisition of such information in the course of authorized investigative activities, the retention of such information, or its dissemination as appropriate to the responsible authorities in other jurisdictions. (AGG-Dom, Part II)

2.9. (U) Use of Classified Investigative Technologies

(U) Inappropriate use of classified investigative technologies may risk the compromise of such technologies. Hence, in an investigation relating to activities in violation of federal criminal law, that does not concern a threat to the national security or foreign intelligence, the use of such technologies must be in conformity with the Procedures for the Use of Classified Investigative Technologies in Criminal Cases. (AGG-Dom, Part V.B.2)

2.10. (U) Application of AGG-Dom and DIOG

(U//FOUO) The AGG-Dom and DIOG apply to all FBI domestic investigations and operations conducted by "FBI employees" such as, but not limited to, applicable support personnel, intelligence analysts, special agents, task force officers, detailees, FBI contractors, and confidential human sources (CHS). All of these "FBI employees" are bound by the AGG-Dom and DIOG. In the DIOG, the use of "FBI employee" implies the use of all personnel descriptions, if not otherwise prohibited by law or policy. For example, if the DIOG states the "FBI employee" is responsible for a particular investigative activity, the supervisor has the flexibility to assign that responsibility to any person bound by the AGG-Dom and DIOG (i.e., agent, intelligence analyst, task force officer), if not otherwise prohibited by law or policy.

(U//FOUO) FBIHQ Division Policy Implementation Guides cannot be less restrictive than the DIOG. Additionally, FBIHQ Division Policy Implementation Guides must comply with the policy contained in the DIOG, unless approval for deviation from the DIOG is reviewed by the General Counsel and approved by the FBI Deputy Director.

3. (U) Core Values, Roles, and Responsibilities

3.1. (U) The FBI's Core Values

(U) The FBI's values do not exhaust the many goals we wish to achieve, but they capsulate them as well as can be done in a few words. The FBI's core values must be fully understood, practiced, shared, vigorously defended, and preserved. The values are:

- (U) Rigorous obedience to the Constitution of the United States
- (U) Respect for the dignity of all those we protect
- (U) Compassion
- (U) Fairness
- (U) Uncompromising personal integrity and institutional integrity
- (U) Accountability by accepting responsibility for our actions and decisions and their consequences
- (U) Leadership, by example, both personal and professional

(U) By observing these core values, we achieve a high level of excellence in performing the FBI's national security and criminal investigative functions as well as the trust of the American people. Rigorous obedience to constitutional principles ensures that individually and institutionally our adherence to constitutional guarantees is more important than the outcome of any single interview, search for evidence, or investigation. Respect for the dignity of all reminds us to wield law enforcement powers with restraint. Fairness and compassion ensure that we treat everyone with the highest regard for constitutional, civil, and human rights. Personal and institutional integrity reinforce each other and are owed to our Nation in exchange for the sacred trust and great authority conferred upon us.

(U) We who enforce the law must not merely obey it. We have an obligation to set a moral example that those whom we protect can follow. Because the FBI's success in accomplishing its mission is directly related to the support and cooperation of those we protect, these core values are the fiber that holds together the vitality of our institution.

(U) Compliance

(U) All FBI personnel must fully comply with all laws, rules, and regulations governing FBI investigations, operations, programs and activities, including those set forth in the AGG-Dom. We cannot and do not countenance disregard for the law for the sake of expediency in anything we do. The FBI expects its personnel to ascertain the laws and regulations that govern the activities in which they engage, to acquire sufficient knowledge of those laws, rules, and regulations to understand their requirements and to conform their professional and personal conduct accordingly. Under no circumstances will expediency justify disregard for the law. Further, the FBI requires its employees to report to proper authority any known or suspected failures to adhere to the law, rules or regulations by themselves or others. Information for reporting such violations is available from the Office of Integrity and Compliance (OIC).

FBI policy must be consistent with Constitutional, legal and regulatory requirements. Additionally, the FBI must provide sufficient training to affected personnel and ensure that appropriate oversight monitoring mechanisms are in place.

3.2. (U) Deputy Director Roles and Responsibilities

(U//FOUO) The Deputy Director is the proponent of the DIOG, and he has oversight regarding compliance with the DIOG and subordinate implementing procedural directives and divisional specific policy implementation guides (PG). The Deputy Director is also responsible for the development and the delivery of necessary training and the execution of the monitoring and auditing processes. The Deputy Director works through the Corporate Policy Office (CPO) to ensure that the DIOG is updated, as necessary, to comply with changes in the law, rules, or regulations, but not later than one year from the effective date of this DIOG, and every thre years thereafter.

3.3. (U) Special Agent/Intelligence Analyst/Task Force Officer/FBI Contractor/Others Roles and Responsibilities

(U//FOUO) Agents, analysts, task force officers (TFO), FBI contractors and others bound by the AGG-Dom and DIOG must:

A. (U//FOUO) Ensure compliance with the DIOG standards for initiating, conducting, and closing an investigative activity; collection activity; or use of an investigative method, as provided in the DIOG;

B. (U//FOUO) Obtain training on the DIOG standards relevant to his/her position and perform activities consistent with those standards;

C. (U//FOUO) Ensure all investigative activity complies with the Constitution, federal law, executive orders, Presidential Directives, AGG-Dom, other Attorney General Guidelines, Treaties, Memoranda of Agreement/Understanding, this policy document, and any other applicable legal and policy requirements (if an agent, analyst, TFO, or other individual is unsure of the legality of any action, he/she must consult with his/her supervisor and Chief Division Counsel [CDC] or OGC);

D. (U//FOUO) Ensure that civil liberties and privacy are protected throughout the assessment or investigative process;

E. (U//FOUO) Conduct no investigative activity solely on the basis of activities that are protected by the First Amendment or solely on the basis of the race, ethnicity, national origin or religion of the subject;

F. (U//FOUO) Comply with the law, rules, or regulations, and report any non-compliance concern to the proper authority, as stated in the DIOG Section 3.1; and

G. (U//FOUO) Identify victims who have suffered direct physical, emotional, or financial harm as result of the commission of federal crimes, offer the FBI's assistance to victims of these crimes and provide victims' contact information to the responsible FBI Victim Specialist, and keep them updated on the status of the investigation. The FBI's responsibility for assisting victims is continuous as long as there is an open investigation.

3.4. (U) Supervisor Roles and Responsibilities

A. (U) **Supervisor Defined:** Supervisors include, but are not limited to, Field Office and FBIHQ personnel including: Supervisory Intelligence Analyst (SIA), Supervisory Special Agent (SSA), Supervisory Senior Resident Agent (SSRA), Unit Chief (UC), Assistant Special Agent in Charge (ASAC), Assistant Section Chief (ASC), Section Chief (SC), Special Agent in Charge (SAC), Deputy Assistant Director (DAD), Assistant Director (AD), Assistant Director in Charge (ADIC), and Executive Assistant Director (EAD).

B. (U) **Supervisor Responsibilities:**

1. (U//FOUO) Anyone in a supervisory role that approves/reviews investigative or collection activity must determine whether the standards for initiating, approving, conducting, and closing an investigative activity, collection activity or investigative method, as provided in the DIOG, are satisfied.

2. (U//FOUO) Supervisors must monitor to ensure that all investigative activity, collection activity and the use of investigative methods comply with the Constitution, federal law, Executive Orders, Presidential Directives, AGG-Dom, other Attorney General Guidelines, Treaties, Memoranda of Agreement/Understanding, this policy document, and any other applicable legal and policy requirements.

   (U//FOUO) Supervisors must obtain training on the DIOG standards relevant to their position and conform their decisions to those standards. Supervisors must also ensure that all subordinates have received the required training on the DIOG standards and requirements relevant to their positions.

   (U//FOUO) All supervisors must ensure that civil liberties and privacy are protected throughout the investigative process.

   (U//FOUO) If encountering a practice that does not comply with the law, rules, or regulations, the supervisor must report that compliance concern to the proper authority and, when necessary, take action to maintain compliance.

   (U//FOUO) Supervisors must not retaliate or take adverse action against persons who raise compliance concerns. (See OIC non-retaliation policy in the CPO policy and guidance library)

C. (U//FOUO) **Supervisory Delegation:** Throughout the DIOG, any requirement imposed on a supervisor may be performed by a designated Acting, Primary or Secondary Relief Supervisor, unless specified otherwise by federal statute, Executive Order, Presidential Directive, Attorney General Guidelines, FBI policy, or any other applicable regulation. All delegations must be made in writing and retained appropriately.

   (U//FOUO) A supervisor may delegate authority to a supervisor one level junior to himself or herself, unless specified otherwise (e.g., the SAC may delegate authority to the ASAC). This delegation must: (i) identify the task delegated; (ii) identify the supervisory position given approval authority; (iii) be in writing; and (iv) be retained appropriately. This delegation authority is not further delegable. Except as provided in the preceding paragraph, an SSA or SIA may not delegate authority.

   (U//FOUO) Any supervisor can request that a supervisor at a higher level approve a particular activity, so long as the higher-level supervisor is in the original approval supervisor's "chain-of-command" (e.g., SSA approval is required to open a preliminary investigation, but the SSA requests that his/her ASAC or SAC approve the preliminary investigation because he/she will be on TDY). Unlike delegations of authority which require written documentation, higher supervisory approval than required by the AGG-Dom or DIOG does not require written authorization.

D. (U//FOUO) **File Reviews:** Full-time supervisors or primary relief supervisors (relief supervisors require SAC approval) must conduct investigative file reviews with their subordinates, as discussed below. Investigative file reviews must be conducted with all agents, Resident Agents, TFOs, analysts, detailees, and FBI contractors as appropriate. Investigative file reviews for probationary agents are recommended every 30 days but must be conducted at least every 60 days.

1. (U//FOUO) **Assessment Justification/File Reviews:** Supervisors must conduct 30-day justification reviews for types 1 and 2 assessments and 90-day file reviews for types 3, 4 and 6 assessments, as required in Section 5 of the DIOG. These justification/file reviews must: (i) evaluate the progress made toward the achievement of the authorized purpose and objective; (ii) ensure activities that occurred in the prior 30/90 days were appropriate; (iii) determine whether it is reasonably likely that information may be obtained that is relevant to the authorized objective, thereby warranting an extension for another 30/90 days; (iv) determine whether adequate predication has been developed to open and/or continues to justify a predicated investigation; and (v) determine whether the assessment should be terminated..

   a. (U//FOUO) **Type 1 and 2 Assessments:** Supervisory justification reviews must be conducted for each 30 day period. Following the end of the 30-day period, the agent, analyst, TFO, detailee or FBI contractor and the supervisor have up to 10 calendar days to complete all aspects of the review and to appropriately document the review, as specified in this section of the DIOG.

   b. (U//FOUO) **Type 3, 4 and 6 Assessments:** Supervisory justification/file reviews must be conducted for each 90 day period. Following the end of each 90 day period, the agent, analyst, TFO, detailee or FBI contractor and the supervisor have up to 30 days to complete all aspects of the review and to appropriately document the review, as specified in this section of the DIOG. Investigative file reviews for probationary FBI employees are recommended every 30 days but must be conducted at least every 60 days.

2. (U//FOUO) **Predicated Investigations:** Supervisory investigative file reviews must be conducted for each 90 day period. Following the end of each 90 day period, the agent, analyst, TFO, detailee or FBI contractor and the supervisor have up to 30 days to complete all aspects of the review and to appropriately document the review, as specified in this section of the DIOG. Investigative file reviews for probationary FBI employees are recommended every 30 days but must be conducted at least every 60 days.

3. (U//FOUO) **General Policy for Justification/File Reviews:** A justification/file review must be: (i) in person or by telephone when necessary (e.g., FBI employee is TDY); (ii) conducted in private; and (iii) noted in the Automated Case Support (ACS) Investigative Case Management Case Review or on the FD-71 or Guardian. Justification/file review documentation must be executed in duplicate, with the subordinate being permitted to

16

retain a copy, and the originals retained by the supervisor in each subordinate's administrative folder until the next inspection. If the subordinate only has applicant cases assigned and is in compliance with FBI deadlines and regulations, the in-person conference may be waived. If the conference is waived, the supervisor will make suitable comments concerning the subordinate's caseload, performance, compliance with FBI deadlines and regulations, and record the fact that no conference was held. The results of the justification/file reviews must be considered when preparing mid-year progress reviews, annual appraisals, and developmental worksheets, except this provision does not apply to TFOs, other agency detailees, or FBI Contractors.

E. (U//FOUO) **Unaddressed Work for Assessments and Full Investigations**

(U//FOUO)

(U//FOUO)

(U//FOUO)

(U//FOUO)

(U//FOUO) The FD-71 provides a mechanism to assign an Assessment to an appropriate Unaddressed Work File, if appropriate. In the FD-71, the Supervisor must select a reason for assigning the matter to the Unaddressed Work File, and choose the appropriate classification. Upon submitting the FD-71, a new Unaddressed Work File will be opened.

3.5.   (U) Chief Division Counsel Roles and Responsibilities

(U//FOUO) The Chief Division Counsel (CDC) must review all assessments and predicated investigations involving sensitive investigative matters as discussed in DIOG Section 10 as well as review the use of particular investigative methods as discussed in Sections 5 and 11 of the DIOG. The primary purpose of the CDC's review is to ensure the legality of the actions proposed. Review, in this context, includes a determination that the investigative activity is: (i) not legally objectionable (i.e., that it is not based solely on the exercise of First Amendment rights or on the race, ethnicity, national origin or religion of the subject; and (ii) founded upon an authorized purpose and/or adequate factual predication and meets the standard specified in the DIOG. The CDC should also include in his or her review and recommendation, if appropriate, a determination of the wisdom of the proposed action (e.g., the CDC may have no legal objection but may recommend denial because the value of the proposal is outweighed by the intrusion into legitimate privacy interests). The CDC's determination that an investigative activity is: (i) not legally objectionable; and (ii) warranted from a mission standpoint is based on facts known at the time of the review and recommendation. Often these facts are not verified or otherwise corroborated until the investigative activity commences. As a result, the CDC may require additional CDC reviews or provide guidance to supervisory personnel with regard to monitoring the results of the investigative activity to ensure that the authorized purpose and/or factual predication remains in tact after the facts are developed.

(U//FOUO) For investigative activities involving a sensitive investigative matter, the CDC must also independently consider the factors articulated in the DIOG and provide the approving authority with a recommendation as to whether, in the CDC's judgment, the investigative activity should be approved. Activities found to be legally objectionable by the CDC may not be approved unless and until the CDC's determination is countermanded by the FBI General Counsel or a delegated designee.

(U//FOUO) Throughout the DIOG, any requirement imposed on the CDC may be performed by an Associate Division Counsel (ADC), Legal Advisor, or designated Acting CDC. All CDC delegations must be made in writing and retained appropriately.

3.6.   (U) Office of the General Counsel Roles and Responsibilities

(U//FOUO) In coordination with the DOJ NSD, the OGC is responsible for conducting regular reviews of all aspects of FBI national security and foreign intelligence activities. The primary purpose of the OGC's review is to ensure the legality of the actions proposed. These reviews, conducted at FBI Field Offices and Headquarters' Units, broadly examine such activities for compliance with the AGG-Dom and other applicable requirements. Review, in this context, includes a determination that the investigative activity is: (i) not legally objectionable (i.e., that it is not based solely on the exercise of First Amendment rights or on the race, ethnicity, national origin or religion of the subject; and (ii) founded upon an authorized purpose and/or adequate factual predication and meets the standard specified in the DIOG. The OGC should also include in its review and recommendation, if appropriate, a determination of the wisdom of the proposed action (e.g., the OGC may have no legal objection but may recommend denial because the value of the proposal is outweighed by the intrusion into legitimate privacy interests). The OGC's determination that an investigative activity is: (i) not legally objectionable; and (ii) warranted from a mission standpoint is based on facts known at the time of the review and recommendation. Often these facts are not verified or otherwise corroborated until the investigative activity commences. As a result, the OGC may require additional OGC reviews or provide guidance to supervisory personnel with regard to monitoring the results of the investigative activity to ensure that the authorized purpose and/or factual predication remains in tact after the facts are developed.

(U//FOUO) For those investigative activities involving a sensitive investigative matter requiring OGC review, the OGC must independently consider the factors articulated in the DIOG and provide the approving authority with a recommendation as to whether, in the OGC's judgment, the investigative activity should be approved.

(U//FOUO) Throughout the DIOG, any requirement imposed on the General Counsel may be delegated and performed by a designated OGC attorney. All delegations must be made in writing and retained appropriately.

3.7.   (U) Corporate Policy Office Roles and Responsibilities

(U//FOUO) Subject to the guidance of the Deputy Director, the CPO has oversight of the implementation of the DIOG. In the process of implementing and analyzing the DIOG, the CPO should report any apparent compliance risk areas directly to the OIC. Additionally, the CPO will work directly with the OIC to ensure that the policies, training and monitoring are adequate to meet compliance monitoring procedures.

3.8.   (U) Office of Integrity and Compliance Roles and Responsibilities

(U//FOUO) OIC is responsible for reviewing the DIOG, and working with each FBI Division and the CPO, to identify compliance risk areas and ensure the adequacy of policy statements, training and monitoring. When compliance risk areas are identified, the OIC works with the Divisions, Field Offices, and/or programs affected by the risk and develops programs to review the adequacy of policy statements, training, and monitoring and mitigates those concerns appropriately.

3.9.   (U) Operational Program Manager Roles and Responsibilities

(U//FOUO) FBIHQ Operation Program Managers must review notices and actions received from FBI Field Offices pursuant to procedures contained in the applicable FBIHQ substantive Division's policy implementation guide. This responsibility includes notifying the appropriate DOJ entity of FBI Field Office and FBIHQ investigative activities, within the time period specified by the AGG-Dom, when required.

(U//FOUO) FBIHQ Operational Program Managers are responsible for identifying, prioritizing, and analyzing potential compliance risks within their programs regarding implementation of the DIOG, and developing mitigation plans where warranted.

(U//FOUO) Operational Program Managers must proactively identify and take appropriate action to resolve potential compliance concerns. In identifying possible compliance concerns, Program Managers should consider the following indicators of possible compliance issues:

A. (U//FOUO) Similar activities being handled differently from Squad-to-Squad / Unit-to-Unit / Field Office-to-Field Office;

B. (U//FOUO) Unusually high need for contact with Headquarters' Division for basic information on how to conduct an activity;

C. (U//FOUO) Apparent confusion over how to conduct a certain activity;

D. (U//FOUO) Conflicting policy;

E. (U//FOUO) Non-existent/inaccurate/wrongly targeted training;

F. (U//FOUO) Monitoring mechanisms that do not exist or do not test the right information (e.g. file reviews/program management); and

G. (U//FOUO) Inadequate audit for compliance.

(U//FOUO) Operational Program Managers may not retaliate or take adverse action against persons who raise compliance concerns.

3.10. (U) Division Compliance Officer Roles and Responsibilities

(U//FOUO) Each FBIHQ Division and Field Office must have a Division Compliance Officer (DCO) who will proactively identify potential non-compliance risk areas concerning the implementation of the DIOG and report them to the proper authority and the OIC. The DCO must always be aware that the focus of a compliance program is the identification and resolution of a compliance problem and the process must not be punitive or retaliatory.

3.11. (U) FBI Headquarters Approval Levels

(U//FOUO) If a DIOG provision does not specifically provide, or prohibit, FBIHQ approval authority for conducting certain investigative activities or investigative methods, the below Field Office approval authorities equate to the following FBIHQ personnel and approving officials when FBIHQ initiates, conducts, or closes an investigative activity or utilizes an investigative method:

- (U//FOUO) Field Office Analyst or Special Agent (SA) = FBIHQ Analyst, SA, or Supervisory Special Agent (SSA);

- (U//FOUO) Field Office Supervisory Intelligence Analysts (SIA) = FBIHQ SIA;

- (U//FOUO) Chief Division Counsel (CDC) = FBIHQ Office of the General Counsel (OGC);

- (U//FOUO) Field Office SSA = FBIHQ Unit Chief (UC); and

- (U//FOUO) Special Agent in Charge (SAC) = FBIHQ Section Chief (SC).

4. (U) Privacy and Civil Liberties, and Least Intrusive Methods

4.1. (U) Civil Liberties and Privacy

A. (U) Overview

(U) The FBI is responsible for protecting the American public, not only from crime and terrorism, but also from incursions into their constitutional rights. Accordingly, all AGG-Dom investigative activities must be carried out with full adherence to the Constitution, federal laws and the principles of civil liberty and privacy.

(U) The FBI has a long-established commitment to protecting the civil liberties of Americans as it investigates threats to national security and public safety. As discussed below, compliance with the FBI's comprehensive infrastructure of legal limitations, oversight and self-regulation effectively ensures that this commitment is honored. Because our ability to achieve our mission requires that we have the trust and confidence of the American public, and because that trust and confidence can be significantly shaken by our failure to respect the limits of our power, special care must be taken by all employees to comply with these limitations.

B. (U) Purpose of Investigative Activity

(U) One of the most important safeguards in the AGG-Dom—one that is intended to ensure that FBI employees respect the constitutional rights of Americans—is the threshold requirement that all investigative activity be conducted for an authorized purpose. Under the AGG-Dom that authorized purpose must be an authorized national security, criminal, or foreign intelligence collection purpose.

(U) Simply stating such a purpose is not sufficient, however, to ensure compliance with this safeguard. It is critical that the authorized purpose not be, or appear to be, arbitrary or contrived; that it be well-founded and well-documented; and that the information sought and the investigative method used to obtain it be focused in scope, time, and manner to achieve the underlying purpose. Furthermore, there are constitutional provisions that set limits on what that purpose may be. It may not be solely to monitor the exercise of rights that are protected by the Constitution, and, equally important, the authorized purpose may not be based solely on race, ethnicity, national origin or religion.

(U) It is important to understand how the "authorized purpose" requirement and these constitutional limitations relate to one another. For example, individuals or groups who communicate with each other or with members of the public in any form in pursuit of social or political causes—such as opposing war or foreign policy, protesting government actions, promoting certain religious beliefs—have a fundamental constitutional right to do so. No investigative activity may be conducted for the sole purpose of monitoring the exercise of these rights. If, however, there exists a well-founded basis to conduct investigative activity for one of the authorized purposes listed above—and that basis is not solely the race, ethnicity, national origin or religion of the participants—FBI employees may assess or investigate these activities, subject to other limitations in the AGG-Dom and the DIOG. In this situation, the investigative activity would not be based solely on Constitutionally-protected conduct or on race, ethnicity, nationality or religion. Finally, although investigative activity would be authorized in this situation, it is important that it be conducted in a manner that does not materially interfere with the ability of the individuals or groups to engage in the exercise of Constitutionally-protected rights.

C. (U) **Oversight and Self-Regulation**

(U) Provisions of the AGG-Dom, other AGG, and oversight from DOJ components are designed to ensure the activities of the FBI are lawful, appropriate and ethical as well as effective in protecting the civil liberties and privacy of individuals in the United States. DOJ and the FBI's Inspection Division, OIC, and OGC, along with every FBI employee, share responsibility for ensuring that the FBI meets these goals.

(U) In the criminal investigation arena, oversight of FBI activities has traditionally come from prosecutors and district courts. Because many national security investigations do not result in prosecutions, other oversight mechanisms are necessary. Various features of the AGG-Dom facilitate the DOJ NSD oversight functions in the national security and foreign intelligence collection areas. Relevant requirements and provisions include: (i) required notification by the FBI to the DOJ NSD concerning a full investigation that involves foreign intelligence collection, a full investigation of a United States person in relation to a threat to the national security; or a national security investigation involving a "sensitive investigative matter;" (ii) an annual report by the FBI to the DOJ NSD concerning the FBI's foreign intelligence collection program, including information reflecting the scope and nature of foreign intelligence collection activities in each FBI Field Office; (iii) access by the DOJ NSD to information obtained by the FBI through national security or foreign intelligence activities; and (iv) general authority for the Assistant Attorney General for National Security to obtain reports from the FBI concerning these activities. (AGG-Dom, Intro.4.C)

(U) The DOJ NSD's Oversight Section and the FBI's OGC are responsible for conducting regular reviews of all aspects of FBI national security and foreign intelligence activities. These reviews, conducted at FBI Field Offices and FBIHQ Divisions, broadly examine such activities for compliance with the AGG-Dom and other applicable requirements.

(U) Further examples of oversight mechanisms include the involvement of both FBI and prosecutorial personnel in the review of undercover operations involving sensitive circumstances; notice requirements for investigations involving sensitive investigative matters; and notice and oversight provisions for enterprise investigations, which involve a broad examination of groups implicated in criminal and national security threats. These requirements and procedures help to ensure that the rule of law is respected in the FBI's activities and that public confidence is maintained in these activities. (AGG-Dom, Intro.4.C)

(U) In addition to the above-mentioned oversight entities DOJ has in place, the FBI is subject to a regime of oversight, legal limitations, and self-regulation designed to ensure strict adherence to civil liberties. This regime is comprehensive and has many facets, including the following:

1. (U) The Foreign Intelligence Surveillance Act of 1978, as amended, and Title III of the Omnibus and Streets Act of 1968. These laws establish the processes for obtaining judicial approval of: electronic surveillance and physical searches for the purposes of collecting foreign intelligence and electronic surveillance for the purpose of collecting evidence of crimes.

2. (U) The Whistleblower Protection Acts of 1989 and 1998: These laws protect whistleblowers from retaliation.

3. (U) The Freedom of Information Act of 1966: The law provides the public with access to FBI documents not covered by a specific statutory exemption.

4. (U) The Privacy Act of 1974: The purpose of the Privacy Act is to balance the government's need to maintain information about United States citizens and legal permanent resident aliens with the rights of those individuals to be protected against unwarranted invasions of their privacy stemming from the government's collection, use, maintenance, and dissemination of that information. The Privacy Act forbids the FBI and other federal agencies from collecting information about how individuals exercise their First Amendment rights, unless that collection is expressly authorized by statute or by the individual, or is pertinent to and within the scope of an authorized law enforcement activity (5 U.S.C. § 552a[e][7]). Except for collection of foreign intelligence, activities authorized by the AGG-Dom are authorized law enforcement activities or activities for which there is otherwise statutory authority for purposes of the Privacy Act. Foreign intelligence collection is not an authorized law enforcement activity.

(U) Congressional Oversight is conducted by various committees of the United States Congress, but primarily by the Judiciary and Intelligence Committees. These committees exercise regular, vigorous oversight into all aspects of the FBI's operations. To this end, the National Security Act of 1947 requires the FBI to keep the intelligence committees (for the Senate and House of Representatives) fully and currently informed of substantial intelligence activities. This oversight has significantly increased in breadth and intensity since the 1970's, and it provides important additional assurance that the FBI conducts its investigations according to the law and the Constitution.

(U) The FBI's counterintelligence and counterterrorism operations are subject to significant self-regulation and oversight beyond that conducted by Congress. The Intelligence Oversight Board (IOB), comprised of members from the President's Intelligence Advisory Board (PIAB), also conducts oversight of the FBI. Among its other responsibilities, the IOB reviews violations of The Constitution, national security law, E.O. or Presidential Decision Directive (PDD) by the FBI and the other intelligence agencies, and issues reports thereon to the President and the Attorney General.

(U) Internal FBI safeguards include: (i) the OGC's Privacy and Civil Liberties Unit (PCLU), which reviews plans of any record system proposed within the FBI for compliance with the Privacy Act and related privacy protection requirements and policies; (ii) the criminal and national security undercover operations review committees, comprised of senior DOJ and FBI officials, which review all proposed undercover operations that involve sensitive circumstances; (iii) the Sensitive Operations Review Committee (SORC), comprised of

b5

; (iv) all FBI employees have an obligation to report violations of the DIOG to their supervisor, other management officials, or appropriate authorities; and (v) the FBI requirement for training of new FBI employees and periodic training for all FBI employees to maintain currency on the latest guidelines, changes to laws and regulations, and judicial decisions related to constitutional rights and liberties.

(U) The AGG-Dom and DIOG set forth the standards and requirements under which an investigative activity may be initiated and are designed to provide FBI employees with a framework that maintains the proper balance between the public's need for effective law enforcement and protection of the national security and the protection of civil liberties and privacy. Among the provisions that specifically serve to protect civil liberties and privacy are the following: (i) the prohibition against initiating investigations based solely on the exercise of First Amendment rights or other constitutionally protected activity; (ii) the requirement that FBI employees use the least intrusive method reasonable under the circumstances to achieve their investigative goals; and (iii) the prohibition against engaging in ethnic and racial profiling. Further, in the context of collecting foreign intelligence, the FBI is further required to operate openly and consensually with United States persons, to the extent practicable.

4.2. (U) Protection of First Amendment Rights

(U) A fundamental principle of the Attorney General's guidelines for FBI investigations and operations since the first guidelines were issued in 1976 has been that investigative activity may not be based solely on the exercise of rights guaranteed by the First Amendment to the United States Constitution. This principle carries through to the present day in the AGG-Dom. There is a corollary to this principle in the Privacy Act of 1974, 5 U.S.C. § 552a, which prohibits the retention of information describing how a person exercises rights under the First Amendment, unless there is a valid law enforcement purpose.

(U) The First Amendment states:

> *(U) Congress shall make no law respecting an establishment of religion or prohibiting the free exercise thereof; or abridging the freedom of speech, or of the press; or of the right of the people to peaceably assemble, and to petition the Government for redress of grievances.*

(U) Although the amendment appears literally to apply only to Congress, the Supreme Court made it clear long ago that it also applies to activities of the Executive Branch, including law enforcement agencies. Therefore, for FBI purposes, it would be helpful to read the introduction to the first sentence as: "The FBI shall take no action respecting . . ." In addition, the word "abridging" must be understood. "Abridging," as used here, means "diminishing." Thus, it is not necessary for a law enforcement action to destroy or totally undermine the exercise of First Amendment rights for it to be unconstitutional; significantly diminishing or lessening the ability of individuals to exercise these rights without an authorized investigative purpose is sufficient.

(U) This is not to say that any diminishment of First Amendment rights is unconstitutional. The Supreme Court has never held that the exercise of these rights is absolute. In fact, the Court has set forth realistic interpretations of what level and kind of government activity actually violates a First Amendment right. For example, taken to an extreme, one could argue that the mere possibility of an FBI agent being present at an open forum (or an on-line presence) would diminish the right of free speech by, for example, an anti-war protestor because he/she would be afraid to speak freely. The Supreme Court, however, has never found an "abridgement" of First Amendment rights based on such a subjective fear. Rather, it requires an action that, from an objective perspective, truly diminishes the speaker's message or his/her ability to deliver it (e.g., pulling the plug on the sound system). For another example, requiring protestors to use a certain parade route may diminish, in a practical sense, delivery of their message. The Court has made it clear, however, that for legitimate reasons (e.g., public safety), the government may impose reasonable limitations in terms of time, place and manner to the exercise of such rights—as long as the ability to deliver the message remains.

(U) While the language of the First Amendment prohibits action that would abridge the enumerated rights, the implementation of that prohibition in the AGG-Dom reflects the Supreme Court's opinions on the constitutionality of law enforcement action that may impact the exercise of First Amendment rights. As stated above, the AGG-Dom prohibits investigative activity for the sole purpose of monitoring the exercise of First Amendment rights. The import of the distinction between this language and the actual text of the First Amendment language is two-fold: (i) the line drawn by the AGG-Dom prohibits even "monitoring" the exercise of First Amendment rights (far short of abridging those rights) as the sole purpose of FBI activity; and (ii) the requirement of an authorized purpose for all investigative activity provides additional protection for the exercise of Constitutionally protected rights.

(U) The AGG-Dom classifies investigative activity that involves a religious or political organization (or an individual prominent in such an organization) or a member of the news media as a "sensitive investigative matter." That designation recognizes the sensitivity of conduct that traditionally involves the exercise of First Amendment rights—i.e., groups who associate for political or religious purposes, and the press. The requirements for opening and pursuing a "sensitive investigative matter" are set forth in Section 10 of this policy document. It should be clear, however, from the discussion below just how pervasive the exercise of First Amendment rights is in American life and that not all protected First Amendment activity will fall within the definition of a "sensitive investigative matter." Therefore, it is essential that FBI employees recognize when investigative activity may have an impact on the exercise of these fundamental rights and be especially sure that any such investigative activity has a valid law nforcement or national security purpose, even if it is not a "sensitive investigative matter" as efined in the AGG-Dom and the DIOG.

(U) Finally, it is important to note that United States persons (and organizations comprised of United States persons) do not forfeit their First Amendment rights simply because they also engage in criminal activity or in conduct that threatens national security. For example, an organization suspected of engaging in acts of domestic terrorism may also pursue legitimate political goals and may also engage in lawful means to achieve those goals. The pursuit of these goals through constitutionally-protected conduct does not insulate them from legitimate investigative focus for unlawful activities—but the goals and the pursuit of their goals through lawful means remain protected from unconstitutional infringement.

(U) When allegations of First Amendment violations are brought to a court of law, it is usually in the form of a civil suit in which a plaintiff has to prove some actual or potential harm. Presbyterian Church v. United States, 870 F.2d 518 (9th Cir. 1989). In a criminal trial, a defendant may seek either or both of two remedies as part of a claim that his or her First Amendment rights were violated: suppression of evidence gathered in the alleged First Amendment violation, a claim typically analyzed under the "reasonableness" clause of the Fourth Amendment, and dismissal of the indictment on the basis of "outrageous government conduct" in violation of the Due Process Clause of the Fifth Amendment.

(U) The scope of each of the primary First Amendment rights and their impact on FBI investigative activity are discussed below. The First Amendment's "establishment clause,"—the prohibition against the government establishing or sponsoring a specific religion—has little application to the FBI and, therefore, is not discussed here.

A. (U) **Free Speech**

(U) The exercise of free speech includes far more than simply speaking on a controversial topic in the town square. It includes such activities as carrying placards in a parade, sending letters to a newspaper editor, posting a web site on the Internet, wearing a tee-shirt with a political message, placing a bumper sticker critical of the President on one's car, and publishing books or articles. The common thread in these examples is conveying a public message or an idea through words or deeds. Law enforcement activity that diminishes a person's ability to communicate in any of these ways may interfere with his or her freedom of speech—and thus may not be undertaken by the FBI solely for that purpose.

(U) The line between constitutionally protected speech and advocacy of violence or of conduct that may lead to violence or other unlawful activity must be understood. In Brandenburg v. Ohio, 395 U.S. 444 (1969), the Supreme Court established a two-part test to determine whether such speech is constitutionally protected: the government may not prohibit advocacy of force or violence except when such advocacy (i) is intended to incite imminent lawless action, and (ii) is likely to do so. Therefore, even heated rhetoric or offensive provocation that could conceivably lead to a violent response in the future is usually protected. Suppose, for example, a politically active group advocates on its web site taking unspecified "action" against persons or entities it views as the enemy, who thereafter suffer property damage and/or personal injury. Under the Brandenburg two-part test, the missing specificity and imminence in the message may provide it constitutional protection. For that reason, law enforcement may take no action that, in effect, blocks the message or punishes its sponsors.

(U) Despite the high standard for prohibiting free speech or punishing those who engage in it, the law does not preclude FBI employees from observing and collecting any of the forms of protected speech and considering its content—as long as those activities are done for a valid law enforcement or national security purpose and conducted in a manner that does not unduly infringe upon the ability of the speaker to deliver his or her message. To be an authorized purpose, it must be one that is authorized by the AGG-Dom—i.e., to further an FBI assessment, predicated investigation, or other authorized function such as providing assistance to other agencies. Furthermore, by following the "Standards for Initiating or Approving an Assessment or Predicated Investigation" as contained in the DIOG, the FBI will ensure that there is a rational relationship between that authorized purpose and the protected speech such that a reasonable person with knowledge of the circumstances could understand why the information is being collected.

(U) Returning to the example posed above, because the group's advocacy of action could be directly related by circumstance to property damage suffered by one of the group's known targets, collecting the speech—although lawfully protected—can lawfully occur. Similarly, listening to the public talks by a religious leader, who is suspected of raising funds for a terrorist organization, may yield clues as to his motivation, plan of action, and/or hidden messages to his followers. FBI employees should not, therefore, avoid collecting First

Amendment protected speech if it is relevant to an authorized AGG-Dom purpose—as long as they do so in a manner that does not inhibit the delivery of the message or the ability of the audience to hear it, and so long as the method of collection is the least intrusive means feasible to gather the relevant information.

(U) In summary, during the course of lawful investigative activities, the FBI may lawfully collect, retain, and consider the content of constitutionally protected speech, so long as: (i) the collection is logically related to an authorized investigative purpose; (ii) the collection does not actually infringe on the ability of the speaker to deliver his or her message; and (iii) the method of collection is the least intrusive alternative feasible.

B. (U) **Exercise of Religion**

(U) Like the other First Amendment freedoms, the "free exercise of religion" clause is broader than commonly believed. First, it covers any form of worship of a deity—even forms that are commonly understood to be cults or fringe sects, as well as the right not to worship any deity. Second, protected religious exercise also extends to dress or food that is required by religious edict, attendance at a facility used for religious practice (no matter how unlikely it appears to be intended for that purpose), observance of the Sabbath, raising money for evangelical or missionary purposes, and proselytizing. Even in controlled environments like prisons, religious exercise must be permitted—subject to reasonable restrictions as to time, place, and manner. Another feature of this First Amendment right is that it is a matter of heightened sensitivity to some Americans—especially to devout followers. For this reason, it is a matter that is more likely to provoke an adverse reaction if the right is violated—regardless of which religion is involved. Therefore, when essential investigative activity may impact this right, it must be conducted in a manner that avoids the actual—and the appearance of—interference with religious practice to the maximum extent possible.

(U) While there must be an authorized purpose for any investigative activity that could have an impact on religious practice, this does not mean religious practitioners or religious facilities are completely free from being examined as part of an assessment or predicated investigation. If such practitioners are involved in—or such facilities are used for—activities that are the proper subject of FBI-authorized investigative or intelligence collection activities, their religious affiliation does not "immunize" them to any degree from these efforts. It is paramount, however, that the authorized purpose of such efforts be properly documented. It is also important that investigative activity directed at religious leaders or at conduct occurring within religious facilities be focused in time and manner so as not to infringe on legitimate religious practice by any individual but especially by those who appear unconnected to the activities under investigation.

(U) Furthermore, FBI employees may take appropriate cognizance of the role religion may play in the membership or motivation of a criminal or terrorism enterprise. If, for example, affiliation with a certain religious institution or a specific religious sect is a known requirement for inclusion in a violent organization that is the subject of an investigation, then whether a person of interest is a member of that institution or sect is a rational and permissible consideration. Similarly, if investigative experience and reliable intelligence reveal that members of a terrorist or criminal organization are known to commonly possess or exhibit a combination of religion-based characteristics or practices (e.g., group leaders state that acts of terrorism are based in religious doctrine), it is rational and lawful to consider such a combination in gathering intelligence about the group—even if any one of these, by itself, would constitute an impermissible consideration. By contrast, solely because prior subjects of an investigation of a particular group were members of a certain religion and they claimed a religious motivation for their acts of crime or terrorism, other members' mere affiliation with that religion, by itself, is not a basis to assess or investigate—absent a known and direct connection to the threat under assessment or investigation. Finally, the absence of a particular religious affiliation can be used by analysts and investigators to eliminate certain individuals from further investigative consideration in those scenarios where religious affiliation is relevant.

C. (U) **Freedom of the Press**

(U) Contrary to what many believe, this well-known First Amendment right is not owned by the news media; it is a right of the American people. The drafters of the Constitution believed that a free press was essential to preserving democracy. Although the news media typically seeks to enforce this right, freedom of the press should not be viewed as a contest between law enforcement or national security, on the one hand, and the interests of news media, on the other.

(U) Freedom of the press includes such matters as reasonable access to news-making events, the making of documentaries, and the posting of "blogs." The news gathering function is the aspect of freedom of the press most likely to intersect with law enforcement and national security investigative activities. Within that category, the interest of the news media in protecting confidential sources and the interest of agencies like the FBI in gaining access to these sources who may have evidence of a crime or national security intelligence often clash. The seminal case in this area is Branzburg v. Hayes, 408 U.S. 665 (1977), in which the Supreme Court held that freedom of the press does not entitle a news reporter to refuse to divulge the identity of his source to a federal grand jury. The Court reasoned that, as long as the purpose of law enforcement is not harassment or vindictiveness against the press, any harm to the news gathering function of the press (by revealing source identity) is outweighed by the need of the grand jury to gather evidence of crime.

(U) Partially in response to Branzburg, the Attorney General has issued regulations that govern the issuance of subpoenas for reporter's testimony and telephone toll records, the arrest of a reporter for a crime related to news gathering, and the interview of a reporter as a suspect in a crime arising from the news gathering process. In addition, an investigation of a member of the news media in his official capacity, the use of a reporter as a source, and posing as a member of the news media are all sensitive circumstances in the AGG-Dom and other applicable AG guidelines.

(U) These regulations are not intended to insulate reporters and other news media from FBI assessments or predicated investigations. They are intended to ensure that investigative activity that seeks information from or otherwise involves members of the news media: is appropriately authorized; is necessary for an important law enforcement or national security objective; is the least intrusive means to obtain the information or achieve the goals; and does not unduly infringe upon the news gathering aspect of the constitutional right to freedom of the press.

D. (U) Freedom of Peaceful Assembly and to Petition the Government for Redress of Grievances

(U) Freedom of peaceful assembly, often called the right to freedom of association, present unique issues for law enforcement agencies, including the FBI. Individuals who gather with others to protest government action, or to rally or demonstrate in favor of, or in opposition to, a social cause sometimes present a threat to public safety either by their numbers, by their actions, by the anticipated response to their message, or by creating an opportunity for individuals or other groups with an unlawful purpose to infiltrate and compromise the legitimacy of the group for their own ends. The right to peaceful assembly includes more than just public demonstrations—it includes, as well, the posting of group web sites on the Internet, recruiting others to a cause, marketing a message, and fund raising. All are protected First Amendment activities if they are conducted in support of the organization or political, religious or social cause.

(U) The right to petition the government for redress of grievances is so linked to peaceful assembly and association that it is included in this discussion. A distinction between the two is that an individual may exercise the right to petition the government by himself whereas assembly necessarily involves others. The right to petition the government includes writing letters to Congress, carrying a placard outside city hall that delivers a political message, recruiting others to one's cause, and lobbying Congress or an executive agency for a particular result.

(U) For the FBI, covert presence or action within associations, also called "undisclosed participation," has the greatest potential to impact this Constitutional right. The Supreme Court addressed this issue as a result of civil litigation arising from one of the many protests against the Vietnam War. In Laird v. Tatum, 408 U.S. 1 (1972), the Court found that the mere existence of an investigative program—consisting of covert physical surveillance in public areas, infiltration of public assemblies by government operatives or sources, and the collection of news articles and other publicly available information—for the purpose of determining the existence and scope of a domestic threat to national security does not, by itself, violate the First Amendment rights of the members of the assemblies. The subjective "chill" to the right to assembly, based on the suspected presence of government operatives, did not by itself give rise to legal "standing" to argue that their constitutional rights had been abridged. Instead, the Court required a showing that the complained-of government action would reasonably deter the exercise of that right.

(U) Since Laird v. Tatum was decided, the lower courts have examined government activity on many occasions to determine whether it gave rise to a "subjective chill" or an "objective deterrent." The basic standing requirement establish by Laird remains unchanged today. The lower courts, however, have often imposed a very low threshold of objective harm to survive dismissal of the case. For example, plaintiffs who have shown a loss of membership in an organization, loss of financial support, loss to reputation and status in the community, and loss of employment by members have been granted standing to sue.

(U) More significant for the FBI than the standing issue has been the lower courts' evaluation of investigative activity into First Amendment protected associations since Laird. The courts have held the following investigative activities to be constitutionally permissible under First Amendment analysis: undercover participation in group activities; physical and video surveillance in public areas; properly authorized electronic surveillance; recruitment and operation of sources; collection of information from government, public, and private sources (with consent); and the dissemination of information for a valid law enforcement purpose. However, these decisions were not reached in the abstract. In every case in which the courts have found government action to be proper, the government proved that it was conducted for an authorized law enforcement or national security purpose and that it was conducted in substantial compliance with controlling regulations. In addition, in approving these techniques, the courts have often considered whether a less intrusive technique was available to the agency, and the courts have balanced the degree of intrusion or impact against the importance of the law enforcement or national security objective.

(U) By contrast, since Laird, the courts have found these techniques to be legally objectionable: initiating an investigation solely on the basis of the groups' social or political agenda (even if the agenda made the group susceptible to subversive infiltration); sabotaging or neutralizing the group's legitimate social or political agenda; disparaging the group's reputation or standing; leading the group into criminal activity that otherwise probably would not have occurred; and undermining legitimate recruiting or funding efforts. In every such case, the court found the government's purpose either was not persuasive, was too remote, or was too speculative to justify the intrusion and the potential harm to the exercise of First Amendment rights.

(U) Once again, the message is clear that investigative activity that involves assemblies or associations of United States persons exercising their First Amendment rights must have an authorized purpose under the AGG-Dom—and one to which the information sought and the technique to be employed are rationally related. Less intrusive techniques should always be explored first and those authorizing such activity (which, as discussed above, will almost always constitute a sensitive investigative matter) should ensure that the investigative activity is focused as narrowly as feasible and that the purpose is thoroughly documented.

4.3. (U) Equal Protection under the Law

A. (U) **Introduction**

(U) The Equal Protection Clause of the United States Constitution provides in part that: "No State shall make or enforce any law which shall . . . deny to any person within its jurisdiction the equal protection of the laws." The Supreme Court and the lower courts have made it clear that it applies as well to the official acts of United States government law enforcement agents.[1] Specifically, government employees are prohibited from engaging in invidious discrimination against individuals on the basis of race, ethnicity, national origin, or religious affiliation. This principle is further reflected and implemented for federal law enforcement in the United States Department of Justice's *Guidance Regarding the Use of Race by Federal Law Enforcement Agencies* (hereinafter "DOJ Guidance").

(U) The DOJ Guidance states that investigative and intelligence collection activities must not be based solely on race, ethnicity, national origin, or religious affiliation. Any such activities that are based solely on such considerations are invidious by definition, therefore,

---

[1] See, e.g., Whren v. United States, 517 U.S. 806 (1996); see also Chavez v. Illinois State Police, 251 F.3d 612 (7th Cir. 2001).

unconstitutional. This standard applies to all investigative and collection activity, including collecting and retaining information, opening cases, disseminating information, and indicting and prosecuting defendants. It is particularly applicable to the retention and dissemination of personally identifying information about an individual—as further illustrated in the examples enumerated below.

(U) The constitutional prohibition against invidious discrimination based on race, ethnicity, national origin or religion is relevant to both the national security and criminal investigative programs of the FBI. National security investigations often have ethnic aspects; members of a foreign terrorist organization may be primarily or exclusively from a particular country or area of the world. Similarly, ethnic heritage is frequently the common thread running through violent gangs or other criminal organizations. It should be noted that this is neither a new nor isolated phenomenon. Ethnic commonality among criminal and terrorist groups has been relatively constant and widespread across many ethnicities throughout the history of the FBI.

B. (U) **Policy Principles**

(U) To ensure that assessment and investigative activities and strategies consider racial, ethnic, national origin and religious factors properly and effectively and to help assure the American public that the FBI does not engage in invidious discrimination, the following policy principles are established.

1. (U) The prohibition against investigative activity based solely on race or ethnicity is not avoided by considering it in combination with other prohibited factors. For example, a person of a certain race engaging in lawful public speech about his religious convictions is not a proper subject of investigative activity based solely on any one of these factors—or by the combination of all three. Before collecting and using this information, a well-founded and authorized investigative purpose must exist as to which any or all of these otherwise prohibited factors is relevant.

   (U) When race or ethnicity is a relevant factor to consider, it should not be the dominant or primary factor. Adherence to this standard will not only ensure that it is never the sole factor—it will also preclude undue and unsound reliance on race or ethnicity in investigative analysis. It reflects the recognition that there are thousands and, in some cases, millions of law abiding people in American society of the same race or ethnicity as those who are the subjects of FBI investigative activity, and it guards against the risk of sweeping some of them into the net of suspicion without a sound investigative basis.

   (U) The FBI will not collect or use behavior or characteristics common to particular racial or ethnic community as investigative factors unless they bear clear and specific relevance to a matter under assessment or investigation. This policy is intended to prevent the potential that collecting ethnic characteristics or behavior will inadvertently lead to individual identification based solely on such matters, as well as to avoid the appearance that the FBI is engaged in ethnic or racial profiling.

C. (U) **Guidance on the Use of Race and Ethnic Identity in Assessments and Predicated Investigations**

(U) Considering the reality of common ethnicity or race among many criminal and terrorist groups, some question how the prohibition against racial or ethnic profiling is to be effectively applied—and not violated—in FBI assessments and predicated investigations. The question arises generally in two contexts: (i) with respect to an individual or a group of individuals; and (ii) with respect to ethnic or racial communities as a whole.

1. (U) **Individual Race or Ethnicity as a Factor**

(U) The DOJ Guidance permits the consideration of ethnic and racial identity information based on specific reporting—such as from an eyewitness. As a general rule, race or ethnicity as an identifying feature of a suspected perpetrator, subject, and in some cases, a victim, is relevant if it is based on reliable evidence or information—not conjecture or stereotyped assumptions. In addition, the DOJ Guidance permits consideration of race or ethnicity in other investigative or collection scenarios if it is relevant. These examples illustrate:

   a. (U) The race or ethnicity of suspected members, associates, or supporters of an ethnic-based gang or criminal enterprise may be collected and retained when gathering information about or investigating the organization.

   b. (U) Ethnicity may be considered in evaluating whether a subject is—or is not—a possible associate of a criminal or terrorist group that is known to be comprised of members of the same ethnic grouping—as long as it is not the dominant factor for focusing on a particular person. It is axiomatic that there are many members of the same ethnic group who are not members of the group; and for that reason, there must be other information beyond race or ethnicity that links the individual to the terrorist or criminal group or to the other members of the group. Otherwise, racial or ethnic identity would be the sole criterion, and that is impermissible

2. (U) **Community Race or Ethnicity as a Factor**

   a. (U) **Collecting and analyzing demographics.** The DOJ guidance and FBI policy permit the FBI to identify locations of concentrated ethnic communities in the Field Office's domain, if these locations will reasonably aid the analysis of potential threats and vulnerabilities, and, overall, assist domain awareness for the purpose of performing intelligence analysis. If, for example, intelligence reporting reveals that members of certain terrorist organizations live and operate primarily within a certain concentrated community of the same ethnicity, the location of that community is clearly valuable—and properly collectible—data. Similarly, the locations of ethnic-oriented businesses and other facilities may be collected if their locations will reasonably contribute to an awareness of threats and vulnerabilities, and intelligence collection opportunities. Also, members of some communities may be potential victims of civil rights crimes and, for this reason, community location may aid enforcement of civil rights laws. Information about such communities should not be collected, however, unless the communities are sufficiently concentrated and established so as to provide a reasonable potential for intelligence collection that would support FBI mission programs (e.g., where identified terrorist subjects from certain countries may relocate to blend in and avoid detection).

(U)   **ethnic/racial demographics.**

c. (U) **General ethnic/racial behavior.** The authority to collect ethnic community location information does not extend to the collection of cultural and behavioral information about an ethnic community that bears no rational relationship to a valid investigative or analytical need. Every ethnic community in the Nation that has been associated with a criminal or national security threat has a dominant majority of law-abiding citizens, resident aliens, and visitors who may share common ethnic behavior but who have no connection to crime or terrorism (as either subjects or victims). For this reason, a broad-brush collection of racial or ethnic characteristics or behavior is not helpful to achieve any authorized FBI purpose and may create the appearance of improper racial or ethnic profiling.

d. (U) **Specific and relevant ethnic behavior.** On the other hand, knowing the behavioral and life style characteristics of known individuals who are criminals or who pose a threat to national security may logically aid in the detection and prevention of crime and threats to the national security within the community and beyond. Focused behavioral characteristics reasonably believed to be associated with a particular criminal or terrorist element of an ethnic community (not with the community as a whole) may be collected and retained. For example, if it is known through intelligence analysis or otherwise that individuals associated with an ethnic-based terrorist or criminal group conduct their finances by certain methods, travel in a certain manner, work in certain jobs, or come from a certain part of their home country that has established links to terrorism, those are relevant factors to consider when investigating the group or assessing whether it may have a presence within a community. It is recognized that the "fit" between specific behavioral characteristics and a terrorist or criminal group is unlikely to be perfect—that is, there will be members of the group who do not exhibit the behavioral criteria as well as persons who exhibit the behaviors who are not members of the group. Nevertheless, in order to maximize FBI mission relevance and to minimize the appearance of racial or ethnic profiling, the criteria used to identify members of the group within the larger ethnic community to which they belong must be as focused and as narrow as intelligence reporting and other circumstances permit. If intelligence reporting is insufficiently exact so that it is reasonable to believe that the criteria will include an unreasonable number of people who are not involved, then it would be inappropriate to use the behaviors, standing alone, as the basis for FBI activity.

(U) **Exploitive ethnic behavior.** A related category of information that can be collected is behavioral and cultural information about ethnic or racial communities that is reasonably likely to be exploited by criminal or terrorist groups who hide within those communities in order to engage in illicit activities undetected. For example, the existence of a cultural tradition of collecting funds from members within the community to fund charitable causes in their homeland at a certain time of the year (and how that is accomplished) would be relevant if intelligence reporting revealed that, unknown to many donors, the charitable causes were fronts for terrorist organizations or that terrorist supporters within the community intended to exploit the unwitting donors for their own purposes.

4.4. (U) Least Intrusive Method

A. (U) **Overview**

(U) The AGG-Dom requires that the "least intrusive" means or method be considered and—if operationally sound and effective—used to obtain intelligence or evidence in lieu of a more intrusive method. This principle is also reflected in Executive Order 12333, which governs the activities of the United States intelligence community. The concept of least intrusive method applies to the collection of all intelligence and evidence. Regarding the collection of foreign intelligence that is not collected as part of the FBI's traditional national security or criminal missions, the AGG-Dom provides that open and overt collection activity must be used with United States persons if feasible.

(U) By emphasizing the use of the least intrusive means to obtain intelligence and evidence, FBI employees can effectively execute their duties while mitigating potential negative impacts on the privacy and civil liberties of all people encompassed within the investigation, including targets, witnesses, and victims. This principle is not intended to discourage FBI employees from seeking relevant and necessary intelligence, information, or evidence, but rather is intended to encourage investigators to choose the least intrusive—but still effective—means from the available options to obtain the material.

(U) This principle is embodied in statutes and DOJ policies on a variety of topics including electronic surveillance, the use of tracking devices, the temporary detention of suspects, and forfeiture. In addition, the concept of least intrusive method can be found in case law as a factor to be considered in assessing the reasonableness of an investigative method in the face of a First Amendment or due process violation claim. See Clark v. Library of Congress, 750 F.2d 89, 94 (D.C. Cir 1984); Alliance to End Repression v. City of Chicago, 627 F. Supp. 1044, 1055 (N.D. Ill. 1985), citing Elrod v. Burns, 427 U.S. 347, 362-3 (1976).

B. (U) **General Approach to Least Intrusive Method Concept**

(U) Applying the concept of least intrusive method to an investigative or intelligence collection scenario is both a logical process and an exercise in judgment. It is logical in the sense that the FBI employee must first determine the relative intrusiveness of the method that would provide information:

1. (U) Relevant to the assessment or predicated investigation;

2. (U) Within the time frame required by the assessment or predicated investigation;

3. (U) Consistent with operational security and the protection of sensitive sources and methods; and

4. (U) In a manner that provides confidence in the accuracy of the information.

(U) Determining the least intrusive method also requires sound judgment because it is clear that the factors discussed above are not fixed points on a checklist. They require careful consideration based on a thorough understanding of investigative objectives and circumstances.

C. (U) **Determining Intrusiveness**

(U) In determining intrusiveness, the primary factor should be the degree of procedural protection that established law and the AGG-Dom provide for the use of the method. Using this factor, search warrants, wiretaps, and undercover operations are very intrusive. By contrast, investigative methods with limited procedural requirements, such as checks of government and commercial data bases and communication with established sources, are less intrusive.

(U) The following guidance is designed to assist FBI personnel in judging the relative intrusiveness of different methods:

1. (U) **Nature of the information sought:** Investigative objectives generally dictate the type of information required and from whom it should be collected. This subpart is not intended to address the situation where the type of information needed and its location are clear so that consideration of alternatives would be pointless. When the option exists, however, to seek information from any of a variety of places, it is less intrusive to seek information from less sensitive and less protected places. Similarly, obtaining information that is protected by a statutory scheme (e.g., financial records) or an evidentiary privilege (e.g., attorney/client communications) is more intrusive than obtaining information that is not so protected. In addition, if there exists a reasonable expectation of privacy under the Fourth Amendment (i.e., private communications), obtaining that information is more intrusive than obtaining information that is knowingly exposed to public view as to which there is no reasonable expectation of privacy.

2. (U) **Scope of the information sought:** Collecting information regarding an isolated event—such as a certain phone number called on a specific date or a single financial transaction—is less intrusive or invasive of an individual's privacy than collecting a complete communications or financial "profile." Similarly, a complete credit history is a more intrusive view into an individual's life than a few isolated credit charges. In some cases, a complete financial and credit profile is exactly what the investigation

35

requires (for example, investigations of terrorist financing or money laundering). If so, FBI employees should not hesitate to use appropriate legal process to obtain such information if the predicate requirements are satisfied. It is also recognized that operational security—such as source protection—may dictate seeking a wider scope of information than is absolutely necessary for the purpose of protecting a specific target or source. When doing so, however, the concept of least intrusive alternative still applies. The FBI may obtain more data than strictly needed, but it should obtain no more data than is needed to accomplish the operational security goal.

3. (U) **Scope of the use of the method:** Using a method in a manner that captures a greater picture of an individual's or a group's activities is more intrusive than using the same method or a different one that is focused in time and location to a specific objective. For example, it is less intrusive to use a tracking device to verify point-to-point travel than it is to use the same device to track an individual's movements over a sustained period of time. Sustained tracking on public highways would be just as lawful but more intrusive because it captures a greater portion of an individual's daily movements. Similarly, surveillance by closed circuit television that checks a discrete location within a discrete time frame is less intrusive than 24/7 coverage of a wider area. For another example, a computer intrusion device that captures only host computer identification information is far less intrusive than one that captures file content.

4. (U) **Source of the information sought:** It is less intrusive to obtain information from existing government sources (such as state, local, tribal, international, or federal partners) or from publicly-available data in commercial data bases, than to obtain the same information from a third party (usually through legal process) that has a confidential relationship with the subject—such as a financial or academic institution. Similarly, obtaining information from a reliable confidential source who is lawfully in possession of the information and lawfully entitled to disclose it (such as obtaining an address from an employee of a local utility company) is less intrusive than obtaining the information from an entity with a confidential relationship with the subject. It is recognized in this category that the accuracy and procedural reliability of the information sought is an important factor in choosing the source of the information. For example, even if the information is available from a confidential source, a grand jury subpoena, national security letter (NSL), ex parte order, or other process may be required in order to ensure informational integrity.

5. (U) **The risk of public exposure:** Seeking information about an individual or group under circumstances that create a risk that the contact itself and the information sought will be exposed to the individual's or group's detriment and/or embarrassment—particularly if the method used carries no legal obligation to maintain silence—is more intrusive than information gathering that does not carry that risk. Interviews with employers, neighbors, and associates, for example, or the issuance of grand jury subpoenas at a time when the investigation has not yet been publicly exposed are more intrusive than methods that gather information covertly. Similarly, interviews of a subject in a discrete location would be less intrusive than an interview at, for example, a place of employment or other location where the subject is known.

(U) There is a limit to the utility of this list of intrusiveness factors. Some factors may be inapplicable in a given investigation and, in many cases, the choice and scope of the

36

method will be dictated wholly by investigative objectives and circumstances. The foregoing is not intended to provide a comprehensive checklist or even an overall continuum of intrusiveness. It is intended instead to identify the factors involved in a determination of intrusiveness and to attune FBI employees to select, within each applicable category, a less intrusive method if operational circumstances permit. In the end, selecting the least intrusive method that will accomplish the objective is a matter of sound judgment. In exercising such judgment, however, consideration of these factors should ensure that the decision to proceed is well founded.

D. (U) **Standard for Balancing Intrusion and Investigative Requirements**

(U) Once an appropriate method and its deployment have been determined, reviewing and approving authorities should balance the level of intrusion against investigative requirements. This balancing test is particularly important when the information sought involves clearly established constitutional, statutory, or evidentiary rights or sensitive circumstances (such as obtaining information from religious or academic institutions or public fora where First Amendment rights are being exercised), but should be applied in all circumstances to ensure that the least intrusive alternative feasible is being utilized.

(U) Balancing the factors discussed above with the considerations discussed below will help determine whether the method and the extent to which it intrudes into privacy or threatens civil liberties is proportionate to the significance of the case and the information sought.

(U) Considerations on the investigative side of the balancing scale include the:

1. (U) Seriousness of the crime or national security threat;

2. (U) Strength and significance of the intelligence/information to be gained;

3. (U) Amount of information already known about the subject or group under investigation; and

4. (U) Requirements of operational security, including protection of sources and methods.

(U) If, for example, the threat is remote, the individual's involvement is speculative, and the probability of obtaining probative information is low, intrusive methods may not be justified, i.e., they may do more harm than good. At the other end of the scale, if the threat is significant and possibly imminent (e.g., a bomb threat), aggressive measures would be appropriate regardless of intrusiveness.

(U) In addition, with respect to the investigation of a group, if the terrorist or criminal nature of the group and its membership is well established (e.g., al Qaeda, Ku Klux Klan, Colombo Family of La Cosa Nostra), there is less concern that pure First Amendment activity is at stake than there would be for a group whose true character is not yet known (e.g., an Islamic charity suspected of terrorist funding) or many of whose members appear to be solely exercising First Amendment rights (anti-war protestors suspected of being infiltrated by violent anarchists). This is not to suggest that investigators should be less aggressive in determining the true nature of an unknown group, which may be engaged in terrorism or other violent crime. Indeed, a more aggressive and timely approach may be in order to determine whether the group is violent or to eliminate it as a threat. Nevertheless, when First Amendment rights are at stake, the choice and use of investigative methods should be focused in a manner that minimizes potential infringement of those rights. Finally, as the investigation progresses and the subject's or group's involvement becomes clear, more intrusive methods may be justified. Conversely, if reliable information emerges refuting the individual's involvement or the group's criminal or terrorism connections, the use of any investigative methods must be carefully evaluated.

(U) Another consideration to be balanced is operational security. Is it likely that if a less intrusive but feasible method were selected, the subject would detect its use and alter his activities—including his means of communication—to thwart the success of the operation. Operational security—particularly in national security investigations—should not be undervalued and may, by itself, justify covert tactics which, under other circumstances, would not be the least intrusive.

E. (U) Conclusion

(U) The foregoing guidance is offered to assist FBI employees in navigating the often unclear course to select the least intrusive investigative method that effectively accomplishes the operational objective at hand. In the final analysis, the choice of method and balancing of the impact on privacy and civil liberties with operational needs is a matter of judgment, based on training and experience. Pursuant to the AGG-Dom, other applicable laws and policies, and this guidance, FBI employees may use any lawful method allowed, even if intrusive, where the intrusiveness is warranted by the threat to the national security or to potential victims of crime and/or the strength of the information indicating its existence.

5. (U) Assessments

5.1. (U) Overview

(U//FOUO) The *Attorney General's Guidelines for Domestic FBI Operations* (AGG-Dom) combine "threat assessments" under the former *Attorney General's Guidelines for FBI National Security Investigations and Foreign Intelligence Collection* and the "prompt and extremely limited checking out of initial leads" under the former *Attorney General's Guidelines on General Crimes, Racketeering Enterprise and Terrorism Enterprise Investigations* into a new investigative category entitled "assessments." All assessments must either be opened in an investigative classification as an assessment file (e.g.,☐☐☐☐☐), placed in a☐☐☐☐ ☐☐☐☐ (e.g.,☐☐☐☐☐☐☐☐Guardian]), or placed in an☐☐☐☐☐ as discussed in greater detail below.

b2
b7E

(U//FOUO) **Note:** In the DIOG, the word "assessment" has two distinct meanings. The AGG-Dom authorizes as an investigative activity an "assessment" which requires an authorized purpose as discussed in this section of the DIOG. The USIC, however, also uses the word "assessment" to describe written intelligence products, as discussed in DIOG Section 15.7.B.

(U) Assessments authorized under the AGG-Dom do not require a particular factual predication but do require an authorized purpose. Assessments may be carried out to detect, obtain information about, or prevent or protect against federal crimes or threats to the national security or to collect foreign intelligence. (AGG-Dom, Part II and Part II.A)

(U//FOUO) Although "no particular factual predication" is required, the basis of an assessment cannot be arbitrary or groundless speculation, nor can an assessment be based solely on the exercise of First Amendment protected activities or on the race, ethnicity, national origin or religion of the subject. Although difficult to define, "no particular factual predication" is less than "information or allegation" as required for the initiation of a preliminary investigation. For example, an assessment may be conducted when there is a basis to know: (i) whether more information or facts are required to determine if there is a criminal or national security threat; and (ii) there is a rational and articulable relationship between the stated authorized purpose of the assessment on the one hand and the information sought and the proposed means to obtain that information on the other. Regardless of whether specific approval or specific documentation is required, an FBI employee should be able to explain the purpose of an assessment and the reason for the methods used to conduct the assessment. Those FBI employees who conduct assessments are responsible for assuring that assessments are not pursued for frivolous or improper purposes and are not based solely on First Amendment activity or on the race, ethnicity, national origin, or religion of the subject of the assessment. (AGG-Dom, Part II)

(U//FOUO) An FBI employee can search historical information already contained within: (i) FBI data systems; (ii) United States Intelligence Community (USIC) systems to which an FBI employee has access (e.g.,☐☐☐☐☐☐☐☐☐☐☐☐☐☐☐☐☐☐☐☐☐ ☐☐☐☐☐☐☐☐☐☐☐☐☐☐☐); (iii) any other United States Government database to which an FBI employee has access; and (iv) the FBI employee can also conduct open-source Internet searches without initiating an assessment (open-source Internet searches do not include any paid-for-service databases such as Lexis-Nexis and Choicepoint), as further discussed in Section 5.6.A.1 and Section 15. The use of such paid-for-service databases requires the initiation of an assessment or predicated investigation. This allows the FBI employee to possibly resolve a

b2
b7E

matter without the need to conduct new investigative activity and open an assessment. Additionally, through analysis of existing information, the FBI employee may produce products that include, but are not limited to, an Intelligence Assessment, Intelligence Bulletin and [   ] If, while conducting analysis, the FBI employee finds a gap in intelligence that is relevant to an authorized FBI activity, the FBI employee can identify the gap for possible development of a "collection requirement." The applicable [   ] (or other [   ] as directed in the DI PG) must be used to document this analysis. See the Directorate of Intelligence (DI) PG for file classification guidance.

b2
b7E

5.2. (U) Purpose and Scope

(U//FOUO) The FBI cannot be content to wait for leads to come in through the actions of others; rather, we must be vigilant in detecting criminal or national security threats to the full extent permitted by law, with an eye towards early intervention and prevention of criminal or national security incidents before they occur. For example, to carry out its central mission of protecting the national security, the FBI must proactively collect information from available sources in order to identify threats and activities and to inform appropriate intelligence analysis. Collection required to inform such analysis will appear as FBI National Collection Requirements and FBI Field Office Collection Requirements. Likewise, in the exercise of its protective functions, the FBI is not constrained to wait until information is received indicating that a particular event, activity or facility has drawn the attention of would-be perpetrators of terrorism. The proactive authority conveyed to the FBI is designed for, and may be used by, the FBI in the discharge of these responsibilities. The FBI may also conduct assessments as part of its special events management responsibilities. (AGG-Dom, Part II)

(U) More broadly, detecting and interrupting criminal activities at their early stages, and preventing crimes from occurring in the first place, is preferable to allowing criminal plots to come to fruition. Hence, assessments may also be undertaken proactively with such objectives as detecting criminal activities; obtaining information on individuals, groups, or organizations of possible investigative interest, either because they may be involved in criminal or national security-threatening activities or because they may be targeted for attack or victimization in such activities; and identifying and assessing individuals who may have value as confidential human sources. (AGG-Dom, Part II).

(U//FOUO) As described in the below-scenarios, assessments may be used when an "allegation or information" or an "articulable factual basis" (the predicates for predicated investigations) concerning crimes or threats to the national security is obtained and the matter can be checked out or resolved through the relatively non-intrusive methods authorized in assessments (use of least intrusive means). The checking of investigative leads in this manner can avoid the need to proceed to more formal levels of investigative activity (predicated investigation), if the results of an assessment indicate that further investigation is not warranted. (AGG-Dom, Part II) Hypothetical fact patterns are discussed below:

A. (U//FOUO) [   ]

b2
b7E

(U//FOUO)[   ] The FBI employee can analyze historical information already contained within: (i) FBI data systems; (ii) USIC systems to which FBI employees have access (e.g[   ]); (iii) any other United States Government database to which an FBI employee has access; and (iv) can conduct open-source Internet searches without initiating an assessment. Open-source Internet searches do not include any paid-for-service databases such as Lexis-Nexis and Choicepoint.[   ]

b2
b7E

(U//FOUO)[   ]

B. (U//FOUO)[   ]

b2
b7E

(U//FOUO)[   ]

C. (U//FOUO)[   ]

(U//FOUO[   ]

b2
b7E

(U//FOUO)[   ]

D. (U//FOUO)[   ]

b2
b7E

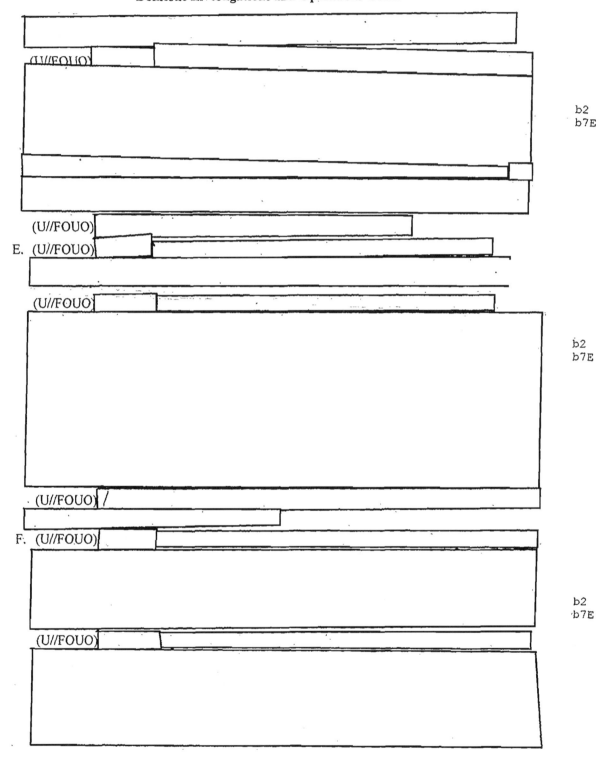

(U//FOUO)

b2
b7E

(U//FOUO)

E. (U//FOUO)

(U//FOUO)

b2
b7E

(U//FOUO)

F. (U//FOUO)

b2
b7E

(U//FOUO)

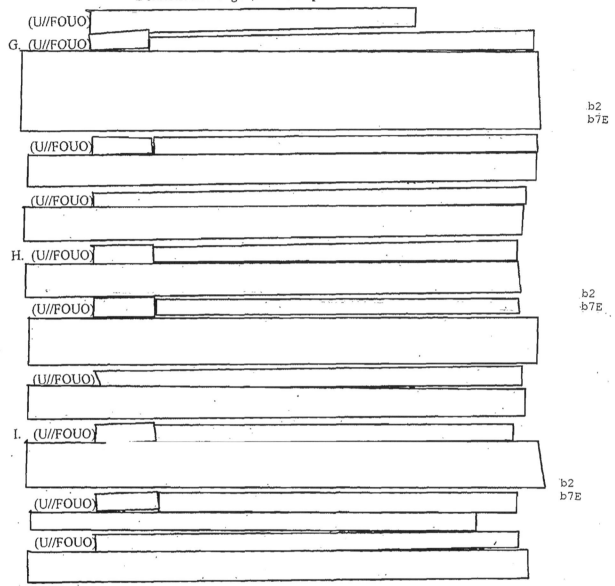

b2
b7E

b2
b7E

b2
b7E

5.3. (U) Civil Liberties and Privacy

(U) The pursuit of legitimate goals without infringing upon the exercise of constitutional freedoms is a challenge that the FBI meets through the application of sound judgment and discretion. In order to ensure that civil liberties are not undermined by the conduct of assessments, every assessment under this subsection must have an authorized purpose and an identified objective. The purpose and objective of the assessment must be documented and retained as described in this section and in DIOG Section 14.

(U) Even when an authorized purpose is present, an assessment could create the appearance that it is directed at or activated by constitutionally protected activity, race, ethnicity, national origin or religion—particularly under circumstances where the link to an authorized FBI mission is not readily apparent. In these situations, it is vitally important that the authorized purpose and the underlying reasons for conducting the assessment and engaging in the proposed methods are well documented.

(U) No investigative activity, including assessments, may be taken solely on the basis of activities that are protected by the First Amendment or on the race, ethnicity, national origin or religion of the subject. If an assessment touches on or is partially motivated by First Amendment activities, race, ethnicity, national origin or religion, it is particularly important to identify and document the basis for the assessment with clarity.

> (U//FOUO) **Example:** Individuals or groups who communicate with each other or with members of the public in any form in pursuit of social or political causes—such as opposing war or foreign policy, protesting government actions, promoting certain religious beliefs, championing particular local, national, or international causes, or a change in government through non-criminal means, and actively recruit others to join their causes— have a fundamental constitutional right to do so. An assessment may not be initiated based solely on the exercise of these First Amendment rights. If, however, a group exercising its First Amendment rights also threatens or advocates violence or destruction of property, an assessment would be appropriate.

(U) The AGG-Dom require that the "least intrusive" means or method be considered and—if operationally sound and effective—used in lieu of more intrusive methods to obtain intelligence and/or evidence. This principle is also reflected in Executive Order 12333, which governs the activities of the USIC. Executive Order 12333 lays out the goals, directions, duties and responsibilities of the USIC. The concept of least intrusive means applies to the collection of all intelligence and evidence, not just that collected by those aspects of the FBI that are part of the intelligence community.

(U) By emphasizing the use of the least intrusive means to obtain intelligence and/or evidence, FBI employees can effectively execute their duties while mitigating the potential negative impact on the privacy and civil liberties and the damage to the reputation of all people encompassed within the investigation or assessment, including targets, witnesses, and victims. This principle is not intended to discourage FBI employees from seeking relevant and necessary intelligence, information, or evidence, but rather is intended to encourage FBI employees to choose the least intrusive—but still effective —means from the available options to obtain the information. (AGG-Dom, Part I.C.2)

5.4. (U) Authorized Purposes (AGG-Dom, Part II.A.2.—Authorized Activities)

A. (U) **Assessment Activities:** During an assessment, the FBI may:

1. (U) Seek information, proactively or in response to investigative leads, relating to activities constituting violations of federal criminal law or threats to the national security;

2. (U) Seek information, proactively or in response to investigative leads, relating to the involvement or role of individuals, groups, or organizations relating to activities constituting violations of federal criminal law or threats to the national security;

3. (U) Identify and obtain information about potential targets of or vulnerabilities to criminal activities in violation of federal law or threats to the national security;

4. (U) Obtain information to inform or facilitate intelligence analysis and planning (AGG-Dom, Part IV);

5. (U) Seek information to identify potential human sources, assess the suitability, credibility, or value of individuals as human sources, validate human sources, or maintain the cover or credibility of human sources, who may be able to provide or obtain information relating to criminal activities in violation of federal law, threats to the national security, or matters of foreign intelligence interest; and

6. (U) Seek information, proactively or in response to investigative leads, relating to matters of foreign intelligence interest responsive to foreign intelligence requirements.

5.5. (U//FOUO) Standards for Initiating or Approving an Assessment

(U//FOUO) Before initiating or approving an assessment, an FBI employee or approving official must determine whether:

A. (U//FOUO) An authorized purpose and objective exists for the conduct of the assessment;

B. (U//FOUO) The assessment is based on factors other than the exercise of First Amendment activities or the race, ethnicity, national origin or religion of the subject; and

C. (U//FOUO) The assessment is an appropriate use of personnel and financial resources.

5.6. (U) Duration, Approval, Notice, Documentation, File Review and Responsible Entity

(U//FOUO) FBIHQ and FBI Field Offices have the authority to conduct all assessment activities as authorized in Section 5.4. Field Office personnel and approving officials, as specified in the DIOG Section 5.6.A.1-6, equate to the following FBIHQ personnel and approving officials when FBIHQ initiates, conducts, or closes an assessment:

- (U//FOUO) Field Office Analyst or Special Agent (SA) = FBIHQ Analyst, SA, or Supervisory Special Agent (SSA);

- (U//FOUO) Field Office Supervisory Intelligence Analysts (SIA) = FBIHQ SIA;

- (U//FOUO) Chief Division Counsel (CDC) = FBIHQ Office of the General Counsel (OGC);

- (U//FOUO) Field Office SSA = FBIHQ Unit Chief (UC); and

- (U//FOUO) Special Agent in Charge (SAC) = FBIHQ Section Chief (SC).

A. (U//FOUO) **Duration, Approval, Notice, Documentation, File Review and Responsible Entity:** An FBI employee must document on the FD-71 or in Guardian the use of or the request and approval for the use of authorized investigative methods in type 1 and 2 assessments (see DIOG Section 5.6.A.1 and 2, below). By exception, certain assessment type 1 and 2 situations may require the use of an electronic communication (EC) to document the use and approval of particular investigative methods. All type 3, 4, and 6 (see DIOG Section 5.6.A.3.4. and 6, below) assessments and authorized investigative methods requiring

45

supervisory approval must use an EC to document the approval of the assessment and the request and approval for the use of an applicable investigative method.

(U//FOUO) For type 5 assessment activities, an FBI employee must follow the duration, approval, and other requirements specified in the FBI's Confidential Human Source Policy Manual (CHSPM), Confidential Human Source Validation Standards Manual (CHSVSM), and *The Attorney General's Guidelines Regarding the Use of FBI Confidential Human Sources* (AGG-CHS), as implemented in⎽⎽⎽⎽. All type 5 assessment activities under this provision must be documented in⎽⎽⎽⎽, unless otherwise directed in the DI PG or other FBIHQ Division PGs. If there is any inconsistency between the CHSPM or CHSVSM and the DIOG, the DIOG controls and OGC should be immediately notified of the conflict.

b2
b7E

(U//FOUO) Listed below are the applicable duration, documentation, justification/file review, approval level, and responsible entity for each type of assessment, described in DIOG Section 5.4 above.

1. (U//FOUO) **Seek information, proactively or in response to investigative leads, relating to activities constituting violations of federal criminal law or threats to the national security** (e.g., the prompt checking of leads on individuals or activity).

   (U//FOUO) **Duration:** There is no time requirement for this type of assessment, but it is anticipated that such assessments will be relatively short. These assessments require recurring 30-day justification reviews by the SSA or SIA as discussed below.

   (U//FOUO) **Documentation:** Guardian will be used for⎽⎽⎽⎽⎽⎽⎽⎽⎽⎽⎽⎽⎽⎽⎽⎽⎽ The electronic FD-71, as discussed below, must be used to⎽⎽⎽⎽⎽⎽⎽⎽⎽⎽⎽⎽⎽⎽⎽⎽⎽⎽⎽⎽⎽⎽ FD-71 or Guardian⎽⎽⎽⎽⎽.

   b2
   b7E.

   . (U//FOUO) **Approval:** An FBI employee may initiate an assessment under this subsection without supervisory approval.⎽⎽⎽⎽⎽⎽⎽⎽⎽⎽⎽⎽⎽⎽⎽ an FD-71 or Guardian⎽⎽⎽⎽⎽⎽⎽⎽⎽⎽⎽⎽⎽⎽⎽⎽⎽⎽ FD-71 or Guardian. The initiation date for this type of assessment is the date the SSA or SIA assigns an FBI employee to conduct the assessment.

   b2
   b7E

   (U//FOUO) As soon as practicable following the determination that this type of assessment involves a sensitive investigative matter, the matter must be brought to the CDC for review and to the SAC for approval to continue the assessment. The term "sensitive investigative matter" is defined in Section 5.7 and Section 10.⎽⎽⎽⎽⎽ the FD-71 or Guardian⎽⎽⎽⎽⎽⎽⎽⎽⎽⎽⎽⎽⎽⎽⎽⎽⎽⎽⎽⎽⎽⎽⎽ Higher supervisory approval, as described in Section 5.9, may be required before using one or more of the following investigative methods: physical surveillance, certain interviews, and tasking of confidential human sources. In addition, as specified in the Division policy implementation guides (PG), there are agreements (e.g., Memoranda

   b2
   b7E

of Agreements/Understanding, Treaties) that may require particular coordination prior to the release/acquisition of federal, state, local, tribal, and foreign government information.

(U//FOUO) **Justification Review:** If this type of assessment is not concluded within 30 days, the SSA or SIA must conduct recurring 30-day justification reviews in accordance with Section 3.4. This justification review must:

a. (U//FOUO) Evaluate the progress made toward achieving the authorized purpose and objective;

b. (U//FOUO) Ensure activities that occurred during the prior 30 days were appropriate;

c. (U//FOUO) Determine whether it is reasonably likely that information will be obtained that is relevant to the authorized objective, thereby warranting an extension for another 30-days;

d. (U//FOUO) Determine whether adequate predication has been developed to justify opening a criminal, counterterrorism, counterintelligence, cyber, or weapons of mass destruction predicated investigation; and

e. (U//FOUO) Determine whether the assessment should be terminated.

(U//FOUO) The FBI employee must ensure that [   ] in the FD-71 or Guardian. The completed FD-71 or Guardian requires supervisory approval before being uploaded. The FD-71 or Guardian must also document supervisory approval for the use of any investigative method that requires approval, such as: physical surveillance; certain interviews; or tasking of confidential human sources (see DIOG Section 5.9). In addition, as specified in the Division PG, there are agreements (e.g., Memoranda of Agreements/Understanding, Treaties) that may require particular coordination prior to the release/acquisition of federal, state, local, tribal and foreign government information. [   ] within the appropriate classification as described in Section 5.14.

b2
b7E

(U//FOUO) **Responsible Entity:** This type of assessment is conducted by the appropriate substantive Field Office Squad.

(U//FOUO) [   ]

(U//FOUO) [   ]

(U//FOUO) [   ]

access, he/she can also review already existing data contained in any United States Government data system and search open source information on the Internet☐ ☐ Open-source Internet searches do not include any paid-for service databases such as Lexis-Nexis and Choicepoint.☐ ☐ If these database checks or open source Internet searches do not reveal any derogatory information, the FBI employee may terminate this activity without opening an assessment or documenting these activities on an FD-71.

(U//FOUO)☐   b2
                                                        b7E

and complete an FD-71.

2. (U//FOUO) **Seek information, proactively or in response to investigative leads, relating to the involvement or role of individuals, groups, or organizations in activities constituting violations of federal criminal law or threats to the national security** (e.g., the prompt checking of leads on groups or organizations).

(U//FOUO) **Duration:** There is no time requirement for this type of assessment, but it is anticipated that such assessments will be relatively short. These assessments require recurring 30-day justification reviews by the SSA or SIA as discussed below.

(U//FOUO) **Documentation:** Guardian☐ The electronic FD-71,☐ FD-71 or   b2
Guardian☐   b7E

(U//FOUO) **Approval:** An FBI employee may initiate an assessment under this subsection without supervisory approval☐ an FD-71 or Guardian☐ the FD-71 or Guardian. The initiation date for this type of assessment is the date the SSA or SIA assigns an FBI employee to conduct the assessment

(U//FOUO) As soon as practicable following the determination that this type of assessment involves a sensitive investigative matter, the matter must be brought to the CDC for review and to the SAC for approval to continue the assessment. The term "sensitive investigative matter" is defined in Section 5.7 and Section 10. When completing the FD-71 or Guardian lead for an assessment involving a sensitive

b2
b7E

Higher supervisory approval, as described in Section 5.9 may be required before using one or more of the following investigative methods: physical surveillance, certain interviews, and tasking of confidential human sources. In addition, as specified in the Division PGs, there are agreements (e.g., Memoranda of Agreements/Understanding, Treaties) that may require particular coordination prior to the release/acquisition of federal, state, local, tribal and foreign government information.

(U//FOUO) **Justification Review:** If this type of assessment is not concluded within 30 days, the SSA or SIA must conduct recurring 30-day justification reviews in accordance with Section 3.4. This justification review must:

a. (U//FOUO) Evaluate the progress made toward achieving the authorized purpose and objective;

b. (U//FOUO) Ensure activities that occurred during the prior 30 days were appropriate;

c. (U//FOUO) Determine whether it is reasonably likely that information will be obtained that is relevant to the authorized objective, thereby warranting an extension for another 30-days;

d. (U//FOUO) Determine whether adequate predication has been developed to justify opening a criminal, counterterrorism, counterintelligence, cyber, or weapons of mass destruction predicated investigation; and

e. (U//FOUO) Determine whether the assessment should be terminated.

(U//FOUO) The FBI employee must ensure that _____ _____ in the FD-71 or Guardian. The completed FD-71 or Guardian requires supervisory approval before being uploaded. The FD-71 or Guardian must also document supervisory approval for the use of any investigative method that requires approval, such as: physical surveillance; certain interviews; or tasking of confidential human sources (see Section 5.9). In addition, as specified in the Division PGs, there are agreements (e.g., Memoranda of Agreements/Understanding, Treaties) that may require particular coordination prior to the release/acquisition of federal, state, local, tribal and foreign government information.

b2
b7E

(U//FOUO) **Responsible Entity:** This type of assessment is conducted by the appropriate substantive Field Office Squad.

(U//FOUO)

b2
b7E

(U//FOUO)

b2
b7E

(U//FOUO)

3. (U) **Identify and obtain information about potential targets of or vulnerabilities to criminal activities in violation of federal law or threats to the national security.**

(U//FOUO) Assessments in this section may include activities designed to collect information for domain analysis that is focused on identifying targets of or vulnerabilities to criminal conduct or threats to the national security. FBIHQ directed National Domain Assessments must be coordinated in advance with the FBIHQ DI, Domain Management Section (DMS). See the DI PG for details.

(U//FOUO) This type of assessment may not be used for the purpose of collecting positive foreign intelligence, although such intelligence may be incidentally collected during this type of assessment. Positive foreign intelligence can only be collected pursuant to Section 5.6.A.6 and Section 9.

b2
b7E

(U//FOUO) **Duration:** An FBI employee may initiate an assessment for this purpose only with prior SSA or SIA approval. The effective date of the assessment is the date the supervisor approves the EC. Such an assessment may continue for as long as necessary to achieve its purpose and objective. When the objective has been met, a closing EC must be approved by the SSA or SIA and uploaded to the file.

(U//FOUO) **Documentation:** The approval to initiate this type of assessment and the request for approval to use applicable investigative methods must be documented in an EC.

(U//FOUO) **Approval:** All assessments conducted pursuant to this subsection must be approved in advance by an SSA or SIA and be opened in either the appropriate [   ] (or other [   ] as directed in the DI PG) or the appropriate substantive investigative classification as an assessment file with an opening EC. The title/case caption of the opening EC must contain the word "Assessment," and the synopsis must identify the purpose and the objective of the assessment. If at the time of the opening, or at anytime thereafter, the assessment involves a sensitive investigative matter, the title/case caption must contain the words "Assessment" and "Sensitive Investigative Matter."

(U//FOUO) **File Review:** This type of assessment requires recurring 90-day file reviews of the assessment file and any sub-file by the SSA or SIA in accordance with Section 3.4.

Investigative file reviews for probationary FBI employees are recommended every 30 days but must be conducted at least every 60 days. This file review must:

a. (U//FOUO) Evaluate the progress made toward achieving the authorized purpose and objective;

b. (U//FOUO) Determine whether it is reasonably likely that information will be obtained that is relevant to the authorized objective, thereby warranting an extension for another 90 days (at least every 60 days for probationary FBI employees);

c. (U//FOUO) Determine whether adequate predication has been developed to justify opening a criminal, counterterrorism, counterintelligence, cyber, or weapons of mass destruction predicated investigation; and

d. (U//FOUO) Determine whether the assessment should be terminated.

(U//FOUO) An SSA or SIA may approve an assessment under this subsection in accordance with the standards listed in the DIOG Section 5.5. However, if the assessment involves a sensitive investigative matter, then the initiation requires prior CDC review and SAC approval. If a sensitive investigative matter arises after the initiation of an assessment, investigative activity must cease until CDC review and SAC approval is acquired. The term "sensitive investigative matter" is defined in Section 5.7 and Section 10. Higher supervisory approval, as described in Section 5.9, may be required prior to use of the following investigative methods: physical surveillance, certain interviews, and tasking of confidential human sources. In addition, as specified in the Division PGs, there are agreements (e.g., Memoranda of Agreements/Understanding, Treaties) that may require particular coordination prior to the release/acquisition of federal, state, local, tribal and foreign government information.

(U//FOUO) Any collection undertaken in order to identify threats, vulnerabilities, or intelligence gaps identified as a result of domain analysis or in response to an FBI National Collection Requirement or FBI Field Office Collection Requirement must be addressed in a separate substantive classification assessment file according to the investigative matter (e.g., [   ]. Additionally, any time an assessment begins to focus on a particular individual, a separate substantive classification assessment file or subfile, as appropriate, according to the investigative matter must be opened on the individual.

b2
b7E

(U//FOUO) **Responsible Entity:** In general, the Field Intelligence Group (FIG) or FBIHQ DI will manage this type of assessment, regardless of whether the assessment is documented in an [   ] (or other [   ] as directed in the DI PG) or a substantive investigative classification file. This includes substantive assessments derived from analysis produced and documented in [   ] (or other [   ] as directed in the DI PG). Under the management of the FIG, substantive Field Office Squads can support the collection of information for this type of assessment. However, substantive Field Office Squads or FBIHQ Units will be responsible for initiating and managing particular kinds of type 3 assessments. These assessments will be documented in the appropriate substantive investigative classification file.

(U//FOUO)

b2
b7E

(U//FOUO)

b2
b7E

(U//FOUO)

b2
b7E

4. (U//FOUO) **Obtain information to inform or facilitate intelligence analysis and planning.** [AGG-Dom, Part IV]

(U//FOUO) Assessments in this section may include activities designed to collect information for domain analysis in order to respond to an FBI National Collection Requirement or FBI Field Office Collection Requirement created in response to FBI operational needs or an intelligence gap identified through strategic analysis that was conducted as part of the FBI's national security or law enforcement responsibilities, as discussed in Sections 5.11 and 5.12. FBIHQ directed National Domain Assessments must be coordinated in advance with the FBIHQ DI, Domain Management Section (DMS). See the DI PG for details.

(U//FOUO) This type of assessment may not be used for the purpose of collecting positive foreign intelligence, although such intelligence may be incidentally collected during this type of assessment. Positive foreign intelligence can only be collected pursuant to Section 5.6.A.6 and Section 9.

(U//FOUO) **Duration:** An FBI employee may initiate an assessment for this purpose only with prior SSA or SIA approval. The effective date of the assessment is the date the supervisor approves the EC. Such an assessment may continue for as long as necessary to achieve its purpose and objective. When the objective has been met, a closing EC must be approved by the SSA or SIA and uploaded to the file.

(U//FOUO) **Documentation:** The approval to initiate this type of assessment and the request for approval to use applicable investigative methods must be documented in an EC. This type of assessment may be documented in either the appropriate [   ] [   ] (or other [   ] as directed in the DI PG) or the appropriate substantive investigative classification assessment file.

b2
b7E

(U//FOUO) **Approval:** All assessments conducted pursuant to this subsection must be approved in advance by an SSA or SIA and be opened in either the appropriate ☐ ☐ (or other ☐ as directed in the DLPG)

b2
b7E

(U//FOUO) **File Review:** This type of assessment requires recurring 90-day file reviews of the assessment file and any sub-file by the SSA or SIA in accordance with DIOG Section 3.4. Investigative file reviews for probationary FBI employees are recommended every 30 days but must be conducted at least every 60 days. This file review must:

a. (U//FOUO) Evaluate the progress made toward achieving the authorized purpose and objective;

b. (U//FOUO) Determine whether it is reasonably likely that information will be obtained that is relevant to the authorized objective, thereby warranting an extension for another 90 days (at least every 60 days for probationary FBI employees);

c. (U//FOUO) Determine whether adequate predication has been developed to justify opening a criminal, counterterrorism, counterintelligence, cyber, or weapons of mass destruction predicated investigation; and

d. (U//FOUO) Determine whether the assessment should be terminated.

(U//FOUO) An SSA or SIA may approve an assessment under this subsection in accordance with the standards listed in the DIOG Section 5.5. However, if the assessment involves a sensitive investigative matter, then the initiation requires prior CDC review and SAC approval. If a sensitive investigative matter arises after the initiation of an assessment, investigative activity must cease until CDC review and SAC approval is acquired. The term "sensitive investigative matter" is defined in Section 5.7 and DIOG Section 10. Higher supervisory approval, as described in Section 5.9, may be required before using the following investigative methods: physical surveillance, certain interviews, and tasking of confidential human sources. In addition, as specified in the Division PGs, there are agreements (e.g., Memoranda of Agreements/Understanding, Treaties) that may require particular coordination prior to the release/acquisition of federal, state, local, tribal and foreign government information.

(U//FOUO) Any collection undertaken in order to identify threats, vulnerabilities, or intelligence gaps identified as a result of domain analysis or in response to an FBI National Collection Requirement or FBI Field Office Collection Requirement must be addressed in a separate substantive classification assessment file according to the investigative matter (e.g., ☐ Additionally, any time an assessment begins to focus on a particular individual, a separate substantive classification assessment file or subfile, as appropriate, according to the investigative matter must be opened on the individual.

b2
b7E

(U//FOUO) **Responsible Entity:** The FIG or FBIHQ DI will manage this type of assessment, regardless of whether the assessment is documented in an [   ] (or other [   ] as directed in the DI PG) or a substantive investigative classification file. This includes substantive assessments derived from analysis produced and documented in [   ] (or other [   ] as directed in the DI PG). Under the management of the FIG, substantive Field Office Squads can support the collection of information in this type of assessment.

b2
b7E

(U//FOUO)[   ]

b2
b7E

(U//FOUO)[   ]

b2
b7E

(U//FOUO)[   ]

b2·
b7E

5. (U//FOUO) **Seek information to identify potential human sources, assess the suitability, credibility, or value of particular individuals as human sources, validate human sources, or maintain the cover or credibility of human sources, who may be able to provide or obtain information relating to criminal activities in violation of federal law, threats to the national security, or matters of foreign intelligence interest.**

(U//FOUO) **Duration:** All such activities must follow the policy requirements established in the FBI's Confidential Human Source Policy Manual (CHSPM), Confidential Human Source Validation Standards Manual (CHSVSM), and *The Attorney General's Guidelines Regarding the Use of FBI Confidential Human Sources* (AGG-CHS), and implemented in [   ] If there is any inconsistency between the CHSPM or

b2
b7E

CHSVSM and the DIOG, the DIOG controls and OGC should be immediately notified of the conflict.

(U//FOUO) **Documentation:** [   ] must be used to document all activities under this provision, unless otherwise directed in the DI PG or other FBIHQ Division PGs.

b2
b7E

(U//FOUO) **Approval:** All approvals must follow the policy requirements established in the FBI's CHSPM, CHSVSM, and the AGG-CHS, and as implemented in [   ].

(U//FOUO) **File Review:** File reviews must be conducted in accordance with the FBI's CHSPM.

(U//FOUO) **Responsible Entity:** A FIG or substantive squad may conduct and manage this type of assessment.

6. (U//FOUO) **Seek information, proactively or in response to investigative leads, relating to matters of foreign intelligence interest responsive to foreign intelligence requirements.**

(U//FOUO) Foreign Intelligence is "information relating to the capabilities, intentions, or activities of foreign governments or elements thereof, foreign organizations, or foreign persons, or international terrorists." The FBI defines a foreign intelligence requirement to be a collection requirement issued by the United States Intelligence Community (USIC) and accepted by the FBI DI. The collection of foreign intelligence pursuant to this definition extends the sphere of the FBI's information-gathering activities beyond federal crimes and threats to the national security, and permits the FBI to seek information regarding a broader range of matters relating to foreign powers, organizations, or persons that may be of interest to the conduct of the United States' foreign affairs. (AGG-Dom, Introduction A.3)

(U//FOUO) Under this authorized purpose, an FBI employee may only collect information that relates to matters of positive foreign intelligence. (See DIOG Section 9 for a description of "positive foreign intelligence.") An FBI employee should prioritize collection against FBI National Collection Requirements before attempting to collect against a positive foreign intelligence requirement. The DI PG furnishes guidance on the prioritization of collection.

(U//FOUO) **Duration:** An FBI employee may initiate an assessment for this purpose only with prior Field Office SSA or SIA approval and FBIHQ Collection Management Section (CMS) approval. The effective date of the assessment is the date FBIHQ CMS approves the assessment. Such an assessment may continue for as long as necessary to achieve its purpose and objectives. When the objective has been met, a closing EC must be approved by the Field Office SSA or SIA and FBIHQ CMS and uploaded to the file.

(U//FOUO) **Documentation:** This type of assessment must use an EC to document the initiation approval of the assessment and the request and approval for the use of applicable investigative methods. Foreign intelligence collected pursuant to this subsection must be maintained in the [   ] or as otherwise determined by FBIHQ CMS. The DI PG further describes this process.

b2
b7E

(U//FOUO) **Approval:** Assessments to collect on matters of "foreign intelligence interest" must be approved in advance by FBIHQ CMS in accordance with the standards listed in Section 5.5.

b2
b7E

In addition to the normal requirement to use the least intrusive method to gather information during an assessment, when conducting this type of assessment the FBI employee must be mindful of the additional requirement to operate openly and consensually with a United States person, to the extent practicable.

(U//FOUO) **File Review:** This type of assessment requires recurring 90-day file reviews of the assessment file and any sub-file by the SSA or SIA in accordance with Section 3.4. Investigative file reviews for probationary FBI employees are recommended every 30 days but must be conducted at least every 60 days. This file review must:

a. (U//FOUO) Evaluate the progress made toward achieving the authorized purpose and objective;

b. (U//FOUO) Determine whether it is reasonably likely that information will be obtained that is relevant to the authorized objective, thereby warranting an extension for another 90 days (at least every 60 days for probationary FBI employees);

c. (U//FOUO) Determine whether adequate predication has been developed to justify opening a criminal, counterterrorism, counterintelligence, cyber, or weapons of mass destruction predicated investigation; and

d. (U//FOUO) Determine whether the assessment should be terminated.

(U//FOUO) If the initiation of the assessment involves a sensitive investigative matter, it must be reviewed by the CDC and approved by the SAC, prior to seeking FBIHQ CMS authorization. If a sensitive investigative matter arises after the initiation of an assessment investigative activity must cease until CDC review and SAC approval is acquired and notice provided to FBIHQ CMS. Higher supervisory approval, as described in Section 5.9, may be required before using the following investigative methods: physical surveillance, certain interviews, and tasking of confidential human sources. In addition, as specified in the Division PGs, there are agreements (e.g., Memoranda of Agreements/Understanding, Treaties) that may require particular coordination prior to the release/acquisition of certain federal, state, local, tribal and foreign government information.

(U//FOUO) Positive foreign intelligence collected pursuant to this subsection must be maintained in [   ] or as otherwise determined by FBIHQ CMS. The title/case caption of the opening EC must contain the word "Assessment," and the synopsis must identify the purpose and the objective of the assessment. If at the time of the opening, or at anytime thereafter, the assessment involves a sensitive investigative matter, the title/case caption must contain the words "Assessment" and "Sensitive Investigative Matter." The DI PG further describes this process.

.b2
b7E

(U//FOUO) **Responsible Entity:** This type of assessment is managed by the FIG and FBIHQ DI.

5.7. (U) Sensitive Investigative Matter / Academic Nexus / Buckley Amendment

A. (U//FOUO) **Sensitive Investigative Matter:** An investigative matter involving the activities of a domestic public official or political candidate (involving corruption or a threat to the national security), religious or political organization or individual prominent in such an organization, or news media, or any other matter which, in the judgment of the official authorizing an investigation, should be brought to the attention of FBI Headquarters and other DOJ officials. (AGG-Dom, Part VII.N.) As a matter of FBI policy, "judgment" means that the decision of the authorizing official is discretionary. DIOG Section 10 and the DIOG classified Appendix G define   b2
                                                                                       b7E

B. (U//FOUO) **Academic Nexus:**   b2
                                                                                       b7E

(U//FOUO) The sensitivity related to an academic institution arises from the American tradition of "academic freedom" (e.g., an atmosphere in which students and faculty are free to express unorthodox ideas and views and to challenge conventional thought without fear of repercussion). Academic freedom does not mean, however, that academic institutions are off limits to FBI investigators in pursuit of information or individuals of legitimate investigative interest.   b2
                                                                                       b7E

(U//FOUO)
                          see the DIOG classified Appendix G.

C. (U//FOUO) **Buckley Amendment:** A request for "academic records" must only be made pursuant to the provisions of the Buckley Amendment (The Family Educational Rights and Privacy Act of 1974, 20 U.S.C. § 1232[g], as amended by Public Law 107-56 ["USA PATRIOT Act"]). An FBI employee is prohibited from receiving "academic records" that have not been properly requested pursuant to the Buckley Amendment. The definition of "academic records" is very broad and covers almost all records about a student other than public, student directory-type information published by the institution. The Buckley   b2
Amendment contains a penalty provision for those institutions that improperly provide   b7E
academic records to law enforcement agencies

(U//FOUO) A Buckley Amendment request for academic records cannot be made during an assessment. In a predicated investigation, a request for academic records must be made pursuant to the Buckley Amendment.

UNCLASSIFIED - FOR OFFICIAL USE ONLY
Domestic Investigations and Operations Guide

5.8. **(U//FOUO) Standards for Initiating or Approving the Use of an Authorized Investigative Method**

(U//FOUO) Prior to initiating or approving the use of an authorized investigative method, an FBI employee or approving official must determine whether:

A. (U//FOUO) The use of the particular investigative method is likely to further an objective of the assessment;

B. (U//FOUO) The investigative method selected is the least intrusive method, reasonable under the circumstances;

C. (U//FOUO) The anticipated value of the assessment justifies the use of the selected investigative method or methods;

D. (U//FOUO) If the purpose of the assessment is to collect positive foreign intelligence, the investigative method complies with the AGG-Dom requirement that the FBI operate openly and consensually with a United States person, to the extent practicable; and

E. (U//FOUO) The method is an appropriate use of personnel and financial resources.

5.9. **(U) Authorized Investigative Methods in Assessments and Predicated Investigations**

(U) The following investigative methods may be used in assessments and predicated investigations:

A. (U) **Obtain publicly available information.** (AGG-Dom, Part II.A.4.a and Part VII.L.)

1. (U) **Scope:** "Publicly available information" is information that is:

   a. (U) Published or broadcast for public consumption;

   b. (U) Available on request to the public;

   c. (U) Accessible on-line or otherwise to the public;

   d. (U) Available to the public by subscription or purchase;

   e. (U) Made available at a meeting open to the public;

   f. (U) Obtained by visiting any place or attending an event that is open to the public; or

   g. (U) Could be seen or heard by any casual observer not involving unconsented intrusion into private places.

   (U//FOUO) [   ]   b2
   [   ]   b7E
   [   ]

2. (U//FOUO) **Approval:** Supervisory approval is not required for use of this method, except as to information gathered at a religious service. Notwithstanding any other policy, tasking a CHS or UCE to attend a religious service during a predicated investigation, whether open to the public or not, requires SSA approval. Tasking a CHS to attend a religious service, whether open to the public or not, during an assessment requires SAC approval.

58
UNCLASSIFIED-FOR OFFICIAL USE ONLY

3. (U//FOUO) **Application:** This investigative method may be used in assessments, national security investigations, criminal investigations, foreign intelligence collection cases, and for assistance to other agencies.

4. (U) **Use/Dissemination:** The use or dissemination of information obtained by this method must comply with the AGG-Dom and DIOG Section 14.

B. (U) **Engage in observation or surveillance not requiring a court order. Surveillance includes physical, photographic and video surveillance where such surveillance does not infringe on a reasonable expectation of privacy and trespass is not required to accomplish the surveillance. (AGG-Dom, Part II.A.4.h)**

1. (U) **Scope**

a. (U//FOUO) **Physical Surveillance Defined:** Physical surveillance is the deliberate observation by an FBI employee of persons, places, or events, on either a limited or continuous basis, in a public or a semi-public (e.g., commercial business open to the public) setting.

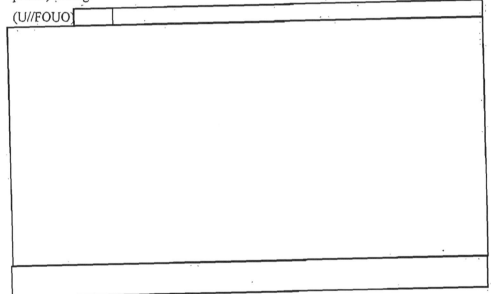

(U//FOUO)

b2
b7E

b. (U//FOUO) **Surveillance Enhancement Devices:** The use of mechanical devices operated by the user (e.g., binoculars; hand-held cameras; radiation, chemical or biological detectors) is authorized in physical surveillance provided that the device is not used to collect information in which a person has a reasonable expectation of privacy (e.g., equipment such as a parabolic microphone or other listening device that would intercept a private conversation or thermal imaging a home is not permitted).

b2
b7E

2. (U//FOUO) **Approval:** During an assessment, physical surveillance may be approved for period of time not to exceed [   ] as explained further below.

. (U//FOUO) **Standards for Initiating or Approving Physical Surveillance During an Assessment:** During an assessment, in addition to the standards contained in Sections 5.5 and 5.8, the FBI employee and supervisor must consider the following:

i. (U//FOUO) Whether the physical surveillance is rationally related to the articulated purpose and objective of the assessment;

ii. (U//FOUO) Whether the physical surveillance is the least intrusive alternative for acquiring needed information;

iii. (U//FOUO) If the physical surveillance is for the purpose of determining a pattern of activity, whether there is a logical nexus between the purpose of the assessment and the pattern of activity he or she is seeking to determine; and

iv. (U//FOUO) If being conducted in order to gather positive foreign intelligence, whether the surveillance is consistent with the requirement that the FBI employee operate openly and consensually with a United States person, to the extent practicable.

b. (U//FOUO)

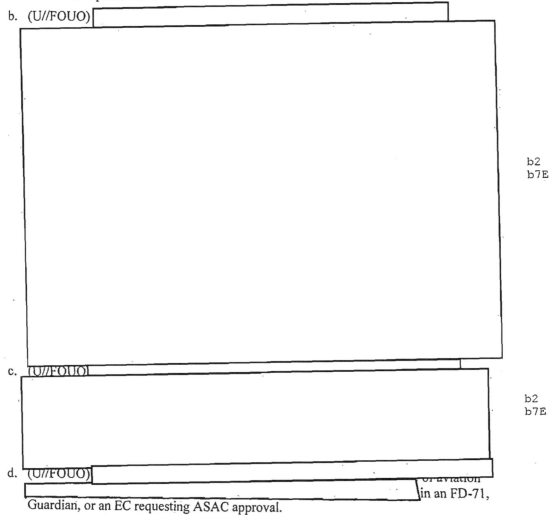

b2
b7E

c. (U//FOUO)

b2
b7E

d. (U//FOUO) _____ or aviation in an FD-71, Guardian, or an EC requesting ASAC approval.

e. (U//FOUO) **Physical Surveillance during Predicated Investigations:** Physical surveillance undertaken during a predicated investigation does not require supervisory approval. [   ]   b2
[   ]   b7E

3. (U//FOUO) **Application:** This investigative method may be used in assessments, national security investigations, criminal investigations, foreign intelligence collection cases, and for assistance to other agencies when it is not otherwise prohibited by AGG-Dom, Part III.B.2-3.

4. (U) **Use/Dissemination:** The use or dissemination of information obtained by this method must comply with the AGG-Dom and DIOG Section 14.

C. (U) **Access and examine FBI and other Department of Justice (DOJ) records, and obtain information from any FBI or other DOJ personnel.** (AGG-Dom, Part II.A.4.b.)

1. (U//FOUO) **Scope:** As part of an assessment or predicated investigation, an FBI employee may access and examine FBI and other DOJ records and may obtain information from any FBI personnel or other DOJ personnel. Access to certain FBI records may be restricted to designated FBI personnel because of the sensitive nature of the information in the record or the classification of the records. These include, but are not limited to: FBI records concerning human source identification; espionage investigations; code word; and other compartmented information.

2. (U//FOUO) **Approval:** Supervisory approval is not required to use this method, except that if the use of records constitutes pattern-based data mining under the Federal Data Mining Reporting Act of 2007, it must be reviewed and approved according to paragraph 3 below.

3. (U//FOUO) **Pattern-Based Data Mining:** The vast majority of data analysis performed during FBI assessments is based on subjects or events and does not meet the definition of pattern-based data mining. Pattern-based data mining is the use of one or more data bases to search for persons who fit a set of group characteristics or patterns of behavior (e.g., the known characteristics of a particular terrorist organization). Any such analysis based solely on racial, ethnic, national origin or religious characteristics is strictly prohibited. Sensitive Operations Review Committee (SORC) approval is required for any analytical search of FBI or other agency data bases that constitute pattern-based data mining, as defined above. Additionally, pursuant to the Federal Data Mining Reporting Act of 2007, the FBI must report all agency initiatives that involve the use of pattern-based data mining to Congress.

4. (U//FOUO) **Application:** This investigative method may be used in assessments, national security investigations, criminal investigations, foreign intelligence collection cases, and for assistance to other agencies.

5. (U) **Use/Dissemination:** The use or dissemination of information obtained by this method must comply with the AGG-Dom and DIOG Section 14.

D. (U) **Access and examine records maintained by, and request information from, other federal, state, local, or tribal, or foreign governmental entities or agencies.** (AGG-Dom, Part II.A.4.c.)

1. (U//FOUO) Scope: As part of an assessment or predicated investigation, an FBI employee may access and examine records maintained by, and request information from, other federal, state, local, or tribal, or foreign governmental entities or agencies. When requesting information using this authority, care must be taken to ensure the entity concerned understands that it is not compelled to provide such information or create a new record for the purpose of assisting the FBI.

2. (U//FOUO) **Approval:** Supervisory approval is not required to use this method for "routine uses," unless such approval is required by Memoranda of Understanding (MOU) or other agreements for requesting such information. The FBI may request another federal agency to disclose Privacy Act-protected records pursuant to the other agency's "routine uses" (5 U.S.C. § 522a[b][3]) or through a written request for a law enforcement purpose (5 U.S.C. § 522a[b][7]). Such written requests (for a law enforcement purpose) pursuant to 5 U.S.C. § 522a(b)(7) may be made by the Director or his designee, provided that such authority may not be delegated below the Section Chief level (28 C.F.R. § 16.40[c]; OMB Guidelines, 40 Fed. Reg. at 28,955). Requests for records or information from a foreign government entity or agency must be appropriately coordinated through the applicable FBI Legat office, Office of International Operations (OIO), INTERPOL, relevant substantive headquarters division, and/or DOJ Office of International Affairs, as necessary. Direct contact is authorized in certain circumstances, such as an imminent threat situation. If the analysis of records obtained in this manner constitutes pattern-based data mining under the Federal Data Mining Reporting Act of 2007, it must be reviewed and approved according to Section 5.9.C.3, above.

   (U//FOUO)

   b2
   b7E

   (U//FOUO) Records received from an outside entity and used during an assessment must be maintained as part of the appropriate file (e.g.,).

3. (U//FOUO) **Application:** This investigative method may be used in assessments, national security investigations, criminal investigations, foreign intelligence collection cases, and for assistance to other agencies.

4. (U) **Use/Dissemination:** The use and/or dissemination of information obtained by this method must comply with the AGG-Dom and DIOG Section 14.

E. (U) **Use online services and resources (whether non-profit or commercial).** (AGG-Dom, Part II.A.4.d.)

1. (U//FOUO) Scope: As part of an assessment or predicated investigation, an FBI employee may use any FBI-approved on-line service or resource that is available by subscription or purchase, including services available only to law enforcement entities.

2. (U//FOUO) **Approval:** Supervisory approval is not required to use this method, although subscribing to or purchasing any new service or resource must be done according to FBI contracting procedures.

   (U//FOUO) **Example:** FBI-approved on-line services or resources include, but are not limited to: Google, Yahoo, or similar Internet search services; data brokers such as ChoicePoint, Westlaw, and Lexis-Nexis; and vehicle, casualty, and property insurance claims databases such as Claim-Search.

3. (U//FOUO) **Application:** This investigative method may be used in assessments, national security investigations, criminal investigations, foreign intelligence collection cases, and for <u>assistance to other agencies</u>.

4. (U) **Use/Dissemination:** The use or dissemination of information obtained by this method must comply with the AGG-Dom and DIOG <u>Section 14</u>.

F. (U) **Interview or request information from members of the public and private entities.** (AGG-Dom, Part II.A.4.f)

1. (U//FOUO) **Scope:** An interview is the questioning of an individual (to include the subject) designed to gather information from the person being interviewed that is accurate, pertinent to, and within the scope of an authorized assessment or predicated investigation. In the normal course of an interview, the FBI employee should divulge the employee's affiliation with the FBI and the true purpose of the interview. Information requested during an interview must be voluntarily provided. If the person who is being interviewed expresses a desire not to provide the information, the FBI employee may not state or imply in any way that the interviewee is compelled to provide information or that adverse consequences may follow if the interviewee does not provide the information. If the person being interviewed indicates he or she wishes to consult an attorney, the interview must immediately stop.

2. (U//FOUO) **Custodial Interviews:** Within the United States, *Miranda* warnings are required to be given prior to custodial interviews if the subject is significantly restricted in his/her freedom of action to a degree normally associated with a formal arrest. For more information refer to the <u>CID</u> and <u>CTD</u> PGs and <u>The FBI Legal Handbook for Special Agents</u> (LHBSA), Section 7-3-2.

3. (U//FOUO) **Approval:** With the exceptions discussed below, interviews do not require supervisory approval.

   a. (U//FOUO) **Contact With Represented Persons:**

   (U//FOUO) CDC review is required before contact with represented persons. Such contact may implicate legal restrictions and affect the admissibility of resulting evidence. Hence, if an individual is known to be represented by counsel in a particular matter, the CDC will follow applicable law and DOJ procedure when reviewing the request to contact the represented individual in the absence of prior notice to counsel. The SAC, CDC, or their designees, and the United States Attorney or their designees must consult periodically on applicable law and DOJ procedure. The Field Office may raise the following issues with the United States Attorney's Office and request that it consult with the DOJ Professional Responsibility Advisory Office, when the issues include, but are not limited to, the inconsistent application of:

(i) state ethics rules; or (ii) rules for contacts with represented persons. (AGG-Dom, Part V.B.1)

b. (U//FOUO) **Members of the United States Congress and their Staffs:**

(U//FOUO) Generally, FBI employees may take information received from congressional offices just as they would take information from other sources, and they may act upon it accordingly.

(U//FOUO) However, prior CDC review, SAC and appropriate FBIHQ AD approval and prior notice to the AD Office of Congressional Affairs (OCA) are required if an investigator seeks to:

b2
b7E

Note: The FBIHQ substantive Division policy implementation guides may contain additional approval/notice requirements.

c. (U//FOUO) **White House Personnel:**

(U//FOUO) CDC review and SAC approval is required before initiating contact with White House personnel. Additionally, CDC review, SAC approval and appropriate FBIHQ Section Chief approval must be obtained prior to conducting an interview of a member of the White House staff. **Note:** The FBIHQ substantive Division policy implementation guides may contain additional approval/notice requirements.

d. (U) **FBIHQ Substantive Division Requirements:**

   i. (U//FOUO) **Counterintelligence Division:** Interviews conducted during counterintelligence assessments and predicated investigations must comply with the requirements contained in the Memorandum of Understanding Between the Department of State and the FBI on Liaison for Counterintelligence Investigations. The FBIHQ Counterintelligence Division PG contains interview approval requirements.

   ii. (U//FOUO) **Other FBIHQ Divisions:** Each FBIHQ Division may provide additional interview approval requirements in its policy implementation guide.

4. (U//FOUO) **Requesting Information Without Revealing FBI Affiliation or the True Purpose of a Request:**

   a. (U//FOUO)

   b. (U//FOUO)

b2
b7E

   c. (U//FOUO)

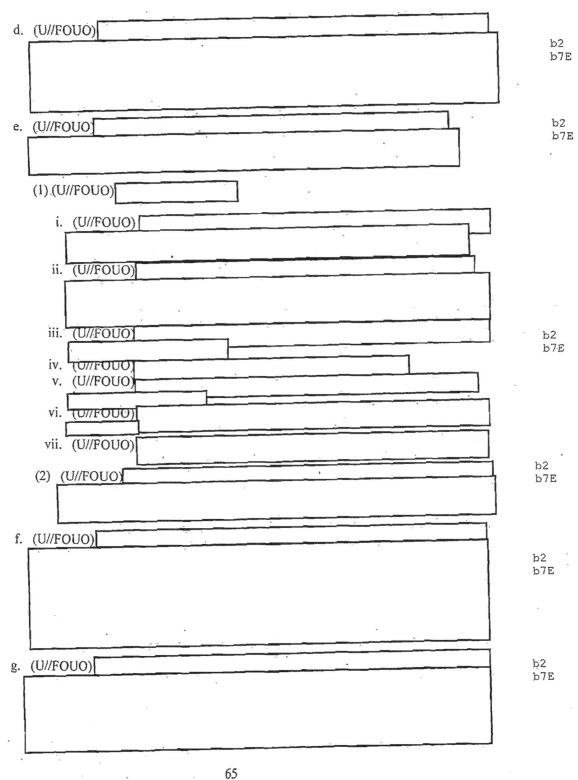

d. (U//FOUO)   b2
                                                                  b7E

e. (U//FOUO)   b2
                                                                  b7E

(1) (U//FOUO)

i.   (U//FOUO)

ii. (U//FOUO)

iii. (U//FOUO)   b2
                                                                  b7E
iv. (U//FOUO)
v.   (U//FOUO)

vi. (U//FOUO)

vii. (U//FOUO)

(2) (U//FOUO)   b2
                                                                  b7E

f. (U//FOUO)   b2
                                                                  b7E

g. (U//FOUO)   b2
                                                                  b7E

b2
b7E

(U//FOUO)

b2
b7E

(U)

i. (U//FOUO)

b2
b7E

ii. (U//FOUO)

b2
b7E

iii. (U//FOUO)

b2
b7E

iv. (U//FOUO)

b2
b7E

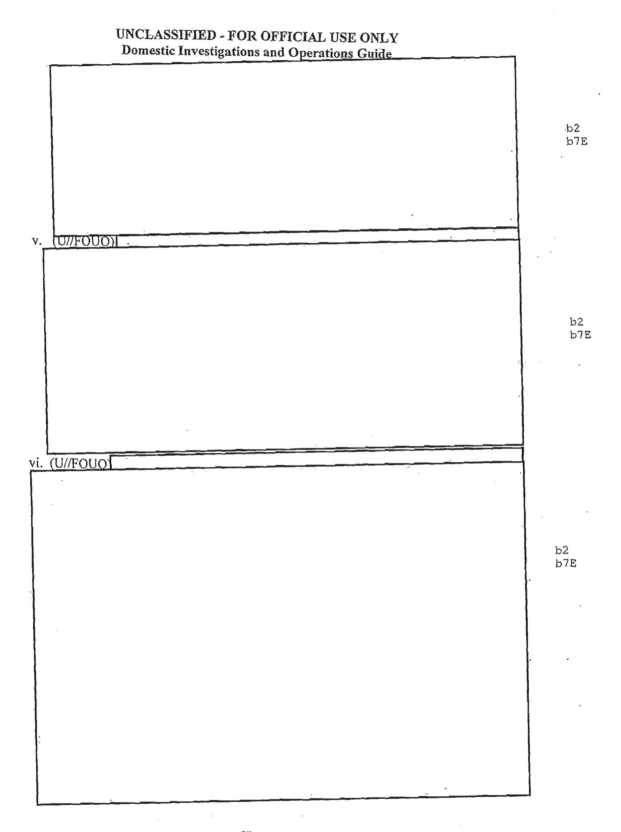

b2
b7E

v. (U//FOUO)

b2
b7E

vi. (U//FOUO)

b2
b7E

vii. (U//FOUO)

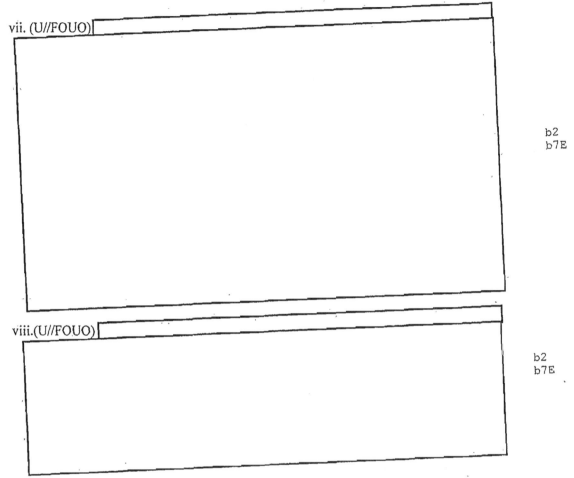

b2
b7E

viii.(U//FOUO)

b2
b7E

5. (U//FOUO) **Application:** This investigative method may be used in assessments, national security investigations, criminal investigations, foreign intelligence collection cases, and for assistance to other agencies when it is not otherwise prohibited by AGG-Dom, Part III.B.2-3.

6. (U) **Use/Dissemination:** The use or dissemination of information obtained by this method must comply with the AGG-Dom and DIOG Section 14.

G. (U) **Accept information voluntarily provided by governmental or private entities.** (AGG-Dom, Part II.A.4.g.)

1. (U//FOUO) **Scope:** As part of an assessment or predicated investigation, an FBI employee may accept information voluntarily provided by federal, state, local, or foreign governmental or private entities to include individuals. Voluntarily provided information includes, but is not limited to, oral as well as documentary and physical evidence such as: a computer hard drive or other electronic media that contains information, paper documents containing information, or physical objects (e.g., handgun or narcotics).

2. (U//FOUO) **Approval:** Supervisory approval is not required to accept voluntarily provided information. Personnel may not request nor knowingly accept information where disclosure would be prohibited by federal law. See, e.g., 18 U.S.C. § 2702 (prohibiting an entity providing electronic communications services from divulging certain communications and other records, except in certain circumstances).

3. (U//FOUO) **Application:** This investigative method may be used in assessments, national security investigations, criminal investigations, foreign intelligence collection cases, and for assistance to other agencies when it is not otherwise prohibited by AGG-Dom, Part III.B.2-3.

4. (U) **Use/Dissemination:** The use or dissemination of information obtained by this method must comply with the AGG-Dom and DIOG Section 14.

H. (U) **Use and recruit human sources in conformity with the Attorney General's Guidelines Regarding the Use of FBI Confidential Human Sources.** (AGG-Dom, Part II.A.4.e)

1. (U//FOUO) The FBI may use and recruit human sources in assessments and predicated investigations in conformity with the AGG-Dom, AGG-CHS, the FBI CHSPM, and the FBI CHSVSM. In this context, "use" means obtaining information from, tasking, or otherwise operating such sources. (AGG-Dom, Part VII.V.)

2. (U//FOUO) A CHS can be "used" in support of an assessment and a predicated investigation or for the purpose of validating, vetting or determining the suitability of another CHS as part of an assessment.

3. (U//FOUO) **Religious Service**—Notwithstanding any other policy, tasking a CHS to attend a religious service, whether or not open to the public, requires SSA approval in a predicated investigation and SAC approval in an assessment.

4. (U//FOUO) All investigative methods should be evaluated to ensure compliance with the admonition that the FBI should use the least intrusive method practicable. That requirement should be particularly observed during an assessment when using a CHS because the use of a CHS during an assessment may be more intrusive than many other investigative methods. Use of a CHS in an assessment should take place only after considering whether there are effective, less intrusive means available to obtain the desired information. The CHS must comply with all constitutional, statutory, and regulatory restrictions and limitations. In addition:

   a. (U//FOUO) CHS use and direction must be limited in focus and scope to what is necessary to accomplish the authorized purpose and objective of the assessment or predicated investigation.

   b2
   b7E

   b. (U//FOUO) A CHS may be directed to seek information about an individual, group or organization only to the extent that such information is necessary to achieve the specific objective of the assessment. If such contact reveals information or facts about an individual, group or organization that meets the requirements of a predicated investigation, a predicated investigation may be opened, as appropriate.

c. (U//FOUO)

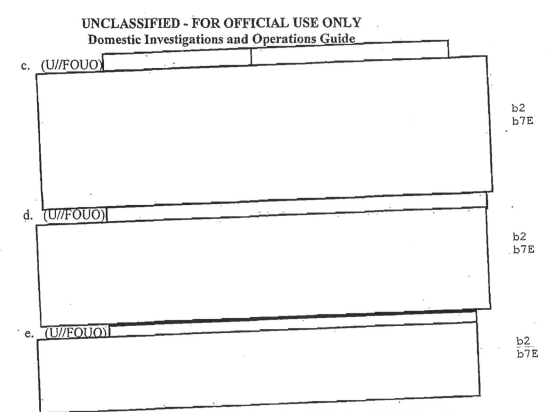

b2
b7E

d. (U//FOUO)

b2
b7E

e. (U//FOUO)

b2
b7E

f. (U//FOUO) If there is any conflict between the CHSPM or CHSVSM and the DIOG, the DIOG controls and OGC should be immediately notified of the conflict.

5. (U//FOUO) **Application:** This investigative method may be used in assessments, national security investigations, criminal investigations, foreign intelligence collection cases, and for <u>assistance to other agencies</u> when it is not otherwise prohibited by AGG-Dom, Part III.B.2.

(U) **Note:** When collecting positive foreign intelligence, the FBI must operate openly and consensually with a United States person, to the extent practicable.

6. (U) **Use/Dissemination:** The use or dissemination of information obtained by this method must comply with the AGG-Dom and DIOG <u>Section 14</u>.

I. (U) **Grand jury subpoenas for telephone or electronic mail subscriber information.** (AGG-Dom, Part II.A.4.i)

1. (U//FOUO) **Scope:** During a type 1 or 2 assessment, an FBI employee may request from an appropriate United States Attorney's Office (USAO) the issuance of a Federal Grand Jury (FGJ) subpoena for the limited purpose of obtaining subscriber information. A FGJ subpoena, under this provision, may not be requested for the purpose of collecting foreign intelligence. For more information regarding FGJ subpoenas, see DIOG <u>Section 11.9</u>.

(U//FOUO) **Note:** The use of Federal Grand Jury Subpoenas, to include subpoenas for telephone or electronic mail subscriber information, is not authorized in a type 3, 4, or 5 assessment or in a type 6 assessment or full investigation initiated for the purpose of collecting positive foreign intelligence.

2. (U//FOUO) **Approval:** In a type 1 or 2 assessment or predicated investigation, supervisory approval is not required prior to requesting a USAO to issue a FGJ subpoena for telephone or electronic mail subscriber information.

3. (U) **Electronic Communications Privacy Act (ECPA) (18 U.S.C. §§ 2701-2712):** ECPA, 18 U.S.C. § 2703 states "a provider of electronic communication service or remote computing service shall disclose to a governmental entity the: (i) name; (ii) address; (iii) local and long distance telephone connection records, or records of sessions, times and durations; (iv) length of service (including start date) and types of service utilized; (v) telephone or instrument number or other subscriber number or identity, including any temporarily assigned network address; and (vi) means and source of payment for such service (including any credit card or bank account number), of a subscriber to or customer of such service when the governmental entity uses . . . a Federal Grand Jury [subpoena]' . . ." (emphasis added)

4. (U//FOUO) **Application:** This investigative method may be used in type 1 and 2 assessments, national security investigations, criminal investigations, and for assistance to other agencies if relevant to an already open type 1 or 2 assessment or predicated investigation. This method may not be used to collect positive foreign intelligence information.

5. (U) **Use/Dissemination:**

b2
b7E

The use or dissemination of information obtained by this method must comply with the AGG-Dom, DIOG Section 14, and the Federal Rules of Criminal Procedure (FRPC) Rule 6.

5.10. (U) Investigative Methods Not Authorized During Assessments

(U) The following methods may not be used in an assessment:

(U//FOUO) **Note:** For use of lawful investigative methods during the recruitment, assessment and validation of a CHS, refer to the AGG-CHS, CHSPM, and CHSVSM.

A. (U) Mail covers

B. (U) Physical searches of personal or real property where a warrant or court order is not legally required because there is no reasonable expectation of privacy (e.g., trash covers)

C. (U) Consensual monitoring of communications, including consensual computer monitoring

D. (U) Use of closed-circuit television, direction finders, and other monitoring devices

E. (U) Polygraph examinations

F. (U) Undercover operations

G. (U//FOUO) Compulsory process, including grand jury subpoenas (except: subscriber information during type 1 and 2 assessments), administrative and other subpoenas, and National Security Letters

H. (U) Accessing stored wire and electronic communications and transactional records

I. (U) Use of pen registers and trap and trace devices

J. (U) Electronic surveillance

K. (U) Physical searches where there is a reasonable expectation of privacy

L. (U) Acquisition of foreign intelligence information in conformity with Title VII of the Foreign Intelligence Surveillance Act (FISA)

5.11.   (U//FOUO) FBI National Collection Requirements

(U//FOUO) The FBIHQ DI establishes FBI National Collection Requirements after coordination with FBIHQ OGC, other FBIHQ substantive Divisions, and Field Offices. An FBI National Collection Requirement describes information needed by the FBI to: (i) identify or obtain information about potential targets of, or vulnerabilities to, federal criminal activities or threats to the national security; or (ii) inform or facilitate intelligence analysis and planning pertinent to the FBI's law enforcement or national security missions.

(U//FOUO)

b2
b7E

(U//FOUO)

(i)   (U//FOUO)

(ii)   (U//FOUO)

b2
b7E

(U//FOUO)

[redacted]

: (U//FOUO) Before any investigative activity is initiated in order to respond to an FBI National Collection Requirement, an assessment must be initiated or already open. An assessment cannot be opened solely based upon an FBI National Collection Requirement. An authorized purpose (national security or criminal threat) must exist and an objective must be clearly articulated that identifies an authorized purpose prior to opening an assessment. During an assessment, the FBI is authorized to collect against any FBI National Collection Requirement that is relevant to the assessment because such requirements are issued for information necessary to identify potential threats or vulnerabilities (e.g., type 3 assessment) or to collect information necessary for intelligence analysis (e.g., type 4 assessment). [redacted]

(U//FOUO) [redacted]

(U//FOUO) [redacted]

5.12. (U//FOUO) FBI Field Office Collection Requirements

(U//FOUO) An FBI Field Office Collection Requirement describes information needed by the field to: (i) identify or obtain information about potential targets of or vulnerabilities to federal criminal activities or threats to the national security; or (ii) inform or facilitate intelligence analysis and planning pertinent to the FBI's law enforcement or national security missions.

(U//FOUO) Before any investigative activity may be conducted to respond to an FBI Field Office Collection Requirement, an assessment must be initiated or already open. An assessment cannot be opened solely based upon an FBI Field Office Collection Requirement [redacted]

The DI PG contains detailed guidance regarding the Field Office Collection Requirements.

5.13. (U) Retention and Dissemination of Privacy Act Records

(U//FOUO) The Privacy Act restricts the maintenance of records relating to the exercise of First Amendment rights by individuals who are United States persons. Such records may be maintained if the information is pertinent to and within the scope of authorized law enforcement activities or for which there is otherwise statutory authority for the purposes of the Privacy Act (5 U.S.C. § 522a[e][7]). Activities authorized by the AGG-Dom are authorized law enforcement activities. Thus, information concerning the exercise of First Amendment rights by United States persons may be retained if it is pertinent to or relevant to the FBI's law enforcement or national security activity. Relevancy must be determined by the circumstances. If the information is not relevant to the law enforcement activity being conducted, then it may not be retained. For more information see DIOG Section 4. (AGG-Dom, Part I.C.5)

(U//FOUO) Even if information obtained during an assessment does not warrant opening a predicated investigation, the FBI may retain personally identifying information for criminal and national security purposes. In this context, the information may eventually serve a variety of valid analytic purposes as pieces of the overall criminal or intelligence picture are developed to detect and disrupt criminal and terrorist activities. In addition, such information may assist FBI personnel in responding to questions that may subsequently arise as to the nature and extent of the assessment and its results, whether positive or negative. Furthermore, retention of such information about an individual collected in the course of an assessment will alert other Divisions or Field Offices considering conducting an assessment on the same individual that the particular individual is not a criminal or national security threat. As such, retaining personally identifying information collected in the course of an assessment will also serve to conserve resources and prevent the initiation of unnecessary assessments and other investigative activities.

(U) **Marking Closed Assessments That Contain Personal Information:** Information obtained during an assessment that has insufficient value to justify further investigative activity may contain personal information. As a result: (i) when records retained in an assessment specifically identify an individual or group whose possible involvement in criminal or national security-threatening activity was checked out through the assessment; and (ii) the assessment turns up no sufficient basis to justify further investigation of the individual or group, then the records must be clearly annotated as follows: "It is noted that the individual or group identified during the assessment does not warrant further FBI investigation at this time. It is recommended that this assessment be closed." Extreme care should be taken when disseminating personally identifiable information collected during an assessment that does not lead to sufficient facts to open a predicated investigation. If personal information from the assessment is disseminated outside the FBI according to authorized dissemination guidelines and procedures, it must be accompanied by the required annotation that the assessment involving this individual or group did not warrant further investigation by the FBI at the time the assessment was closed.

b2
b7E

Moreover, an FBI employee, who shares information from such a closed assessment file, must ensure that the specific annotation (as discussed above) is included with the shared information.

5.14. (U) Assessment File Records Management and Retention

(U//FOUO)

b2
b7E

b2
b7E

[redacted] Records must be retained according to National Archives and Records Administration (NARA) regulations.

(U//FOUO) [redacted] The retention of records in Guardian, or any successor information technology system, must be retained according to NARA regulations.

(U//FOUO) Assessments that require prior supervisory approval must have [redacted]

b2
b7E

[redacted] must be approved by the SSA or SIA [redacted] If additional objectives arise during the assessment, they must be [redacted] approved by the SSA or SIA, and [redacted] Assessment classification files must be retained according to NARA regulations.

6. (U) Preliminary Investigations

6.1. (U) Overview

(U) The AGG-Dom authorizes a second level of investigative activity—predicated investigations. Predicated investigations that concern federal crimes or threats to the national security are subdivided into preliminary investigations and full investigations. Preliminary investigations may be initiated on the basis of any "allegation or information" indicative of possible criminal activity or threats to the national security.

6.2. (U) Purpose and Scope

(U//FOUO) Preliminary investigations may be carried out to detect, obtain information about, or prevent or protect against federal crimes or threats to the national security. However, a preliminary investigation cannot be initiated or used solely for the purpose of collecting against Positive Foreign Intelligence Requirements, or for conducting enterprise investigations. Intelligence responsive to Positive Foreign Intelligence Requirements, FBI National Collection Requirements and FBI Field Office Collection Requirements may be collected incidental to a preliminary investigation concerning another person, organization, or entity. If Positive Foreign Intelligence Requirement, FBI National Collection Requirement or FBI Field Office Collection Requirement information is incidentally collected in a preliminary investigation, it should be forwarded to the FIG for evaluation and potential dissemination against collection requirements.

(U) In preliminary investigations, the immediate objectives include such matters as: determining whether a federal crime has occurred or is occurring, or if planning or preparation for such a crime is taking place; identifying, locating, and apprehending the perpetrators; obtaining evidence needed for prosecution; or identifying threats to the national security.

(U) The investigation of threats to the national security may constitute an exercise of the FBI's criminal investigation authority as well as its authority to investigate threats to the national security. As with criminal investigations, detecting and solving crimes and arresting and prosecuting the perpetrators are likely objectives of investigations relating to threats to the national security. These investigations, however, serve important purposes outside the ambit of normal criminal investigations, by providing the basis for decisions concerning other measures needed to protect the national security.

6.3. (U) Civil Liberties and Privacy

(U) The pursuit of legitimate investigative goals without infringing upon the exercise of constitutional freedoms is a challenge that the FBI meets through the application of sound judgment and discretion. In order to further ensure that civil liberties are not undermined by the conduct of criminal and national security investigations, every preliminary investigation under this subsection must have an identified authorized purpose and adequate predication.

(U) No investigative activity, including preliminary investigations, may be taken solely on the basis of activities that are protected by the First Amendment or on the race, ethnicity, national origin or religion of the subject. Preliminary investigations of individuals, groups or organizations must focus on activities related to the threats and or crimes being investigated, not solely on First Amendment activities or on the race, ethnicity, national origin or religion of the subject. In this context, it is particularly important clearly to identify and document the law enforcement or national security basis of the preliminary investigation.

> (U) **Example:** Individuals or groups who communicate with each other or with members of the public in any form in pursuit of social or political causes—such as opposing war or foreign policy, protesting government actions, promoting certain religious beliefs, championing particular local, national, or international causes, or a change in government through non-criminal means, and actively recruit others to join their causes—have a fundamental constitutional right to do so. A preliminary investigation may not be initiated based solely on the exercise of these First Amendment rights.

(U) The AGG-Dom present investigators with a number of authorized investigative methods in the conduct of a preliminary investigation. Considering the effect on the privacy and civil liberties of individuals and the potential to damage the reputation of individuals, some of these investigative methods are more intrusive than others. The least intrusive method feasible is to be used, but the FBI must not hesitate to use any lawful method consistent with the AGG-Dom. A more intrusive method may be warranted in light of the seriousness of a criminal or national security threat.

(U) By emphasizing the use of the least intrusive means to obtain intelligence and/or evidence, FBI employees can effectively execute their duties while mitigating the potential negative impact on the privacy and civil liberties of all people encompassed within the investigation, including targets, witnesses, and victims. This principle is not intended to discourage FBI employees from seeking relevant and necessary intelligence, information, or evidence, but rather is intended to encourage FBI employees to choose the least intrusive—but still effective means—from the available options to obtain the material.

6.4. (U) Legal Authority

A. (U) **Criminal Investigations**

(U) The FBI has statutory authority to investigate all federal crime not assigned exclusively to another federal agency. (See 28 U.S.C. § 533; 18 U.S.C. § 3052; 28 C.F.R. § 0.85 [1])

(U) The FBI also has special investigative jurisdiction to investigate violations of state law in limited circumstances. Specifically, the FBI has jurisdiction to investigate felony killings of state law enforcement officers (28 U.S.C. § 540), violent crimes against interstate travelers (28 U.S.C. § 540A), and serial killers (28 U.S.C. § 540B). Authority to investigate these matters is contingent on receiving a request by an appropriate state official.

B. (U) **Threats to the National Security**

(U) The FBI has authority to investigate threats to the national security pursuant to executive orders, Attorney General authorities, and various statutory sources. (See E.O. 12333; 50 U.S.C. §§ 401 et seq.; 50 U.S.C. §§ 1801 et seq.)

(U) "Threats to the national security" are specifically defined to mean: international terrorism; espionage and other intelligence activities, sabotage, and assassination, conducted by, for, or on behalf of foreign powers, organizations, or persons; foreign computer intrusion; and other matters determined by the Attorney General, consistent with Executive Order 12333 or any successor order. (AGG-Dom, Part VII.S)

6.5. (U) Predication

(U) A preliminary investigation may be initiated on the basis of "information or an allegation" indicating the existence of a circumstance described as follows:

A. (U) An activity constituting a federal crime or a threat to the national security has or may have occurred, is or may be occurring, or will or may occur and the investigation may obtain information relating to the activity or the involvement or role of an individual, group, or organization in such activity. (AGG-Dom, Part II.B.3)

B. (U) An individual, group, organization, entity, information, property, or activity is or may be a target of attack, victimization, acquisition, infiltration, or recruitment in connection with criminal activity in violation of federal law or a threat to the national security and the investigation may obtain information that would help to protect against such activity or threat. (AGG-Dom, Part II.B.3)

(U//FOUO)

 (i) (U//FOUO)

 (ii) (U//FOUO)

b2
b7E

6.6. (U//FOUO) Standards for Initiating or Approving a Preliminary Investigation

(U) Before initiating or approving the conduct of a preliminary investigation, an FBI employee or approving official must determine whether:

A. (U//FOUO) An authorized purpose and adequate predication exist for initiating a preliminary investigation;

B. (U//FOUO) The preliminary investigation is not based solely on the exercise of First Amendment activities or on the race, ethnicity, national origin or religion of the subject; and

C. (U//FOUO) The preliminary investigation is an appropriate use of personnel and financial resources.

6.7. (U) Duration, Approval, Notice, Documentation and File Review

A. (U//FOUO) **Initiation:** The purpose of and predication for a preliminary investigation must be documented in the initiating EC. The effective date of the preliminary investigation is the date the final approval authority (e.g., SSA or SAC) approves the EC.

 1. (U//FOUO) The initiation of a preliminary investigation by the Field Office requires prior approval of the SSA. FBIHQ Division policy implementation guides may require written notification to the appropriate FBIHQ Unit and Section. The initiation of a preliminary investigation does not require FBIHQ and DOJ notification unless the preliminary investigation involves a sensitive investigative matter as discussed in paragraph 3, below.

2. (U//FOUO) The initiation of a preliminary investigation by FBIHQ requires prior approval of the Unit Chief with written notification to the applicable Field Office. The initiation of a preliminary investigation does not require DOJ notification unless the preliminary investigation involves a sensitive investigative matter as discussed in paragraph 3, below.

3. (U//FOUO) **Sensitive Investigative Matter:** The initiation of a preliminary investigation involving a <u>sensitive investigative matter</u>:

   a. (U//FOUO) **Initiated by a Field Office:** requires CDC review, SAC approval, and written notification to the appropriate FBIHQ Unit Chief and Section Chief. Additionally, written notification must be made by the Field Office to the United States Attorney or by the appropriate FBIHQ Section to the DOJ Criminal Division or NSD as soon as practicable but in all events no later than 30 calendar days after the initiation of such an investigation.

   b2
   b7E

   cease until CDC review and SAC approval is acquired and notice is furnished as specified above.

   b. (U//FOUO) **Initiated by FBIHQ:** requires OGC review, Section Chief approval, and written notification to the United States Attorney and the appropriate Field Office or the DOJ Criminal Division or NSD as soon as practicable but in all events no later than 30 calendar days after the initiation of such an investigation.

   must cease until OGC review and Section Chief approval is acquired and notice is furnished as specified above. (AGG-Dom, Part II.B.5.a)

4. (U//FOUO) The Executive Assistant Director (EAD) for the National Security Branch must notify the Deputy Attorney General if FBI Headquarters disapproves a Field Office's initiation of a preliminary investigation relating to a threat to the national security on the ground that the predication for the investigation is insufficient, and the EAD for the National Security Branch is responsible for establishing a system that will allow for the prompt retrieval of such denials. (AGG-Dom, Part II.B.5.d)

B. (U//FOUO) **Extension:** A preliminary investigation must be concluded within six months of its initiation but may be extended for up to six months by the SAC. This extension authority may <u>not</u> be delegated by the SAC to the ASAC. Extensions of preliminary investigations beyond a year are discouraged and may only be approved by the appropriate FBIHQ Unit and Section for "good cause." (AGG-Dom, Part II.B.4.a.ii) **Note:**

b2
b7E

(U//FOUO) The following factors must be used to determine if "good cause" exists to extend the preliminary investigation beyond one year:

- (U//FOUO) Whether logical investigative steps have yielded information that tends to inculpate or exculpate the subject;

- (U//FOUO) The progress that has been made toward determining whether a full investigation should be opened or the preliminary investigation should be closed;

- (U//FOUO) Whether, based on the planned course of investigation for the following six months, it is reasonably likely that information will be obtained that will lead to predication for a full investigation, thereby warranting an extension for another six months, or will lead to exculpatory information, thereby warranting closing the preliminary investigation; and

- (U//FOUO) Whether adequate predication has been developed to justify opening a full investigation or whether sufficient information has been developed that justify closing the preliminary investigation.

C. (U//FOUO) **Closing:** When closing a preliminary investigation, the Field Office or FBIHQ will provide the reason for closing the investigation. When closing a preliminary investigation, the SSA or Unit Chief must ensure that all pending investigative methods have been completed/terminated (e.g., mail covers and pen register/trap and trace).

1. (U//FOUO) Closing a preliminary investigation initiated by a Field Office requires approval from the SSA.

2. (U//FOUO) Closing a preliminary investigation initiated by FBIHQ requires approval from the Unit Chief and notification to the appropriate Field Office.

3. (U//FOUO) Closing a preliminary investigation initiated by a Field Office involving a sensitive investigative matter requires approval from the SAC

4. (U//FOUO) Closing a preliminary investigation initiated by FBIHQ involving a sensitive investigative matter requires approval from the Section Chief

b2
b7E

D. (U//FOUO) **Conversion:** When converting a preliminary investigation to a full investigation, see Section 7 for approval and notification requirements.

E. (U//FOUO) **File Review:** Supervisory file reviews must be conducted at least once every 90 days in accordance with Section 3.4. File reviews for probationary FBI employees must be conducted at least every 60 days.

6.8.   (U//FOUO) Standards for Initiating or Approving the Use of an Authorized Investigative Method

(U//FOUO) Prior to initiating or approving the use of an investigative method, an FBI employee or approving official must determine whether:

A. (U//FOUO) The use of the particular investigative method is likely to further the purpose of the preliminary investigation;

B. (U//FOUO) The investigative method selected is the least intrusive method, reasonable under the circumstances; and

80

C. (U//FOUO) The method to be used is an appropriate use of personnel and financial resources.

6.9. (U) Authorized Investigative Methods in Preliminary Investigations

A. (U) All lawful methods may be used in a preliminary investigation, except for mail opening, physical search requiring a Federal Rules of Criminal Procedure (FCRP) Rule 41 search warrant or a FISA order, electronic surveillance requiring a judicial order or warrant, or Title VII FISA requests. Authorized methods include, but are not limited to, those listed below. Some of the methods listed are subject to special restrictions or review or approval requirements. (AGG-Dom, Part V.4.A)

B. (U//FOUO) A complete discussion of the investigative methods, including approval requirements, is contained in Sections 5 and 11. The use or dissemination of information obtained by the use of the below methods must comply with the AGG-Dom and DIOG Section 14.

   1. (U) Obtain publicly available information.

   2. (U) Access and examine FBI and other DOJ records, and obtain information from any FBI or other DOJ personnel.

   3. (U) Access and examine records maintained by, and request information from, other federal, state, local, or tribal, or foreign governmental entities or agencies.

   4. (U) Use online services and resources (whether non-profit or commercial).

   5. (U) Use and recruit human sources in conformity with the AGG-CHS.

   6. (U) Interview or request information from members of the public and private entities.

   7. (U) Accept information voluntarily provided by governmental or private entities.

   8. (U) Engage in observation or surveillance not requiring a court order.

   9. (U) Grand Jury Subpoenas for telephone or electronic mail subscriber information (see also number 16, below).

  10. (U) Mail covers. (AGG-Dom, Part V.A.2)

  11. (U) Physical searches of personal or real property where a warrant or court order is not legally required because there is no reasonable expectation of privacy (e.g., open fields, trash covers). (AGG-Dom, Part V.A.3)

  12. (U) Consensual monitoring of communications, including consensual computer monitoring, subject to legal review by the CDC or the FBI OGC. When a sensitive monitoring circumstance is involved, the monitoring must be approved by the DOJ Criminal Division or, if the investigation concerns a threat to the national security, by the DOJ NSD. (AGG-Dom, Part V.A.4) Sensitive monitoring circumstances include:

     a. (U) Investigation of a member of Congress, a federal judge, a member of the Executive Branch at Executive Level IV or above, or a person who has served in such capacity within the previous two years (Executive Level I through IV are defined in 5 U.S.C. §§ 5312-5315);

     b. (U) Investigation of the Governor, Lieutenant Governor, or Attorney General of any state or territory, or a judge or justice of the highest court of any state or territory, concerning an offense involving bribery, conflict of interest, or extortion related to the performance of official duties;

c. (U) A party to the communication is in the custody of the Bureau of Prisons or the United States Marshal Service or is being or has been afforded protection in the Witness Security Program; or

d. (U) The Attorney General, the Deputy Attorney General, or an Assistant Attorney General has requested that the FBI obtain prior approval for the use of consensual monitoring in a specific investigation. (AGG-Dom, Part VII.A and O)

(U//FOUO) **Note:** See classified appendix for additional information.

(U//FOUO)

b2
b7E

13. (U) Use of closed-circuit television, direction finders, and other monitoring devices, subject to legal review by the CDC or the FBI OGC. (The methods described in this paragraph usually do not require a court order or warrant unless they involve an intrusion into an area where there is a reasonable expectation of privacy or non-consensual monitoring of communications, but legal review is necessary to ensure compliance with all applicable legal requirements.) (AGG-Dom, Part.V.A.5)

14. (U) Polygraph examinations. (AGG-Dom, Part V.A.6)

15. (U) Undercover operations. In investigations relating to activities in violation of federal criminal law that do not concern threats to the national security or foreign intelligence, undercover operations must be carried out in conformity with *The Attorney General's Guidelines on Federal Bureau of Investigation Undercover Operations*. Investigations that are not subject to the preceding sentence because they concern threats to the national security or foreign intelligence undercover operations involving religious or political organizations must be reviewed and approved by FBI Headquarters, with participation by the DOJ NSD in the review process. (AGG-Dom, Part V.A.7)

16. (U) Compulsory process as authorized by law, including grand jury subpoenas and other subpoenas. National Security Letters (15 U.S.C. §§ 1681u, 1681v; 18 U.S.C. § 2709; 12 U.S.C. § 3414[a][5][A]; 50 U.S.C. § 436), and FISA orders for the production of tangible things. (50 U.S.C. §§ 1861-63). (AGG-Dom, Part V.A.8)

17. (U) Accessing stored wire and electronic communications and transactional records in conformity with chapter 121 of title 18, United States Code (18 U.S.C. §§ 2701–2712). (AGG-Dom, Part V.A.9)

18. (U) Use of pen registers and trap and trace devices in conformity with chapter 206 of title 18, United States Code (18 U.S.C. §§ 3121-3127) or FISA (50 U.S.C. §§ 1841-1846). (AGG-Dom, Part V.A.10)

6.10. (U) Sensitive Investigative Matter / Academic Nexus / Buckley Amendment

(U//FOUO) The title/case caption of the opening or subsequent EC for a preliminary investigation involving a sensitive investigative matter must contain the words "Sensitive Investigative Matter." DIOG Section 10 contains the required approval authority and factors for consideration when determining whether to initiate or approve a predicated investigation involving a sensitive investigative matter.

A. (U//FOUO) **Sensitive Investigative Matter:** An investigative matter involving the activities of a domestic public official or political candidate (involving corruption or a threat to the national security), religious or political organization or individual prominent in such an organization, or news media, or any other matter which, in the judgment of the official authorizing an investigation, should be brought to the attention of FBI Headquarters and other DOJ officials. (AGG-Dom, Part VII.N.) As a matter of FBI policy, "judgment" means that the decision of the authorizing official is discretionary. DIOG Section 10 and/or the DIOG classified Appendix G define

b2
b7E

B. (U//FOUO) **Academic Nexus:**

b2
b7E

(U//FOUO) The sensitivity related to an academic institution arises from the American tradition of "academic freedom" (e.g., an atmosphere in which students and faculty are free to express unorthodox ideas and views and to challenge conventional thought without fear of repercussion). Academic freedom does not mean, however, that academic institutions are off limits to FBI investigators in pursuit of information or individuals of legitimate investigative interest.

(U//FOUO)

see the DIOG classified Appendix G.

b2
b7E

C. (U//FOUO) **Buckley Amendment:** Although not a sensitive investigative matter, a request for "academic records" must only be made pursuant to the provisions of the Buckley Amendment (The Family Educational Rights and Privacy Act of 1974, 20 U.S.C. § 1232[g], as amended by Public Law 107-56 ["USA PATRIOT Act"]). An FBI employee is prohibited from receiving "academic records" that have not been properly requested pursuant to the Buckley Amendment. The definition of "academic records" is very broad and covers almost all records about a student other than public, student directory-type information published by the institution. The Buckley Amendment contains a penalty provision for those institutions that improperly provide academic records to law enforcement agencies

b2
b7E

A Buckley Amendment request for academic records cannot be made during an assessment. In a predicated investigation, a request for academic records must be made pursuant to the Buckley Amendment.

6.11. (U) Program Specific Investigative Requirements

(U//FOUO) Because of the many investigative programs within the FBI, a single universal requirement will not adequately address every program. To facilitate compliance within an existing program, the FBI employee should consult the relevant program policy guidance.

7. (U) Full Investigations

7.1. (U) Overview

(U//FOUO) The AGG-Dom authorizes a second level of investigative activity—predicated investigations. Predicated investigations that concern federal crimes or threats to the national security are subdivided into preliminary investigations and full investigations. Full investigations may be initiated if there is an "articulable factual basis" of possible criminal or national threat activity, as discussed in greater detail in Section 7.5, below. There are three types of full investigations: (i) single and multi-subject; (ii) enterprise; and (iii) positive foreign intelligence collection.

7.2. (U) Purpose and Scope

(U) Full investigations may be initiated to detect, obtain information about, or prevent or protect against federal crimes or threats to the national security or to collect foreign intelligence.

(U) The objective of a full investigation includes: determining whether a federal crime is being planned, prepared for, occurring or occurred; identifying, locating, and apprehending the perpetrators; obtaining evidence for prosecution; identifying threats to the national security; investigating an enterprise (as defined in DIOG Section 8); or collecting positive foreign intelligence.

(U) The investigation of threats to the national security can be investigated under both the FBI's criminal investigation authority and its authority to investigate threats to the national security. As with criminal investigations, detecting and solving crimes, gathering evidence and arresting and prosecuting the perpetrators are frequently the objectives of investigations relating to threats to the national security. These investigations also serve important purposes outside the ambit of normal criminal investigations, however, by providing the basis for decisions concerning other measures needed to protect the national security.

(U//FOUO)

b2
b7E

(U//FOUO) A full investigation solely for the collection of positive foreign intelligence extends the sphere of the FBI's information gathering activities beyond federal crimes and threats to the national security and permits the FBI to seek information regarding a broader range of matters relating to foreign powers, organizations, or persons that may be of interest to the conduct of the United States' foreign affairs. (See DIOG Section 9)

7.3. (U) Civil Liberties and Privacy

(U) The pursuit of legitimate investigative goals without infringing upon the exercise of constitutional freedoms is a challenge that the FBI meets through the application of sound judgment and discretion. In order to further ensure that civil liberties are not undermined by the conduct of criminal and national security investigations, every full investigation under this subsection must have an identified authorized purpose and adequate predication.

(U) No investigative activity, including full investigations, may be taken solely on the basis of activities that are protected by the First Amendment or on the race, ethnicity, national origin or religion of the subject. Full investigations of individuals, groups or organizations must focus on activities related to the threats or crimes being investigated, not solely on First Amendment activities or on the race, ethnicity, national origin or religion of the subject. In this context, it is particularly important clearly to identify and document the law enforcement or national security basis of the full investigation.

> (U) **Example:** Individuals or groups who communicate with each other or with members of the public in any form in pursuit of social or political causes—such as opposing war or foreign policy, protesting government actions, promoting certain religious beliefs, championing particular local, national, or international causes, or a change in government through non-criminal means, and actively recruit others to join their causes—have a fundamental constitutional right to do so. A full investigation may not be initiated based solely on the exercise of these First Amendment rights.

(U) The AGG-Dom authorize all lawful investigative methods in the conduct of a full investigation. Considering the effect on the privacy and civil liberties of individuals and the potential to damage the reputation of individuals, some of these investigative methods are more intrusive than others. The least intrusive method feasible is to be used, but the FBI must not hesitate to use any lawful method consistent with the AGG-Dom. A more intrusive method may be warranted in light of the seriousness of a criminal or national security threat or the importance of a foreign intelligence requirement.

(U) By emphasizing the use of the least intrusive means to obtain intelligence or evidence, FBI employees can effectively execute their duties while mitigating the potential negative impact on the privacy and civil liberties of all people encompassed within the investigation, including targets, witnesses, and victims. This principle is not intended to discourage FBI employees from seeking relevant and necessary intelligence, information, or evidence, but rather is intended to encourage FBI employees to choose the least intrusive—but still effective means—from the available options to obtain the material.

(U) Because the authority to collect positive foreign intelligence enables the FBI to obtain information pertinent to the United States' conduct of its foreign affairs, even if that information is not related to criminal activity or threats to the national security, the information gathered may concern lawful activities. The FBI must accordingly operate openly and consensually with a United States person to the extent practicable when collecting positive foreign intelligence that does not concern criminal activities or threats to the national security.

7.4. (U) Legal Authority

A. (U) Criminal Investigations

(U) The FBI has statutory authority to investigate all federal crime not assigned exclusively to another federal agency. (See 28 U.S.C. § 533; 18 U.S.C. § 3052; 28 C.F.R. § 0.85 [1].)

(U) The FBI also has special investigative jurisdiction to investigate violations of state law in limited circumstances. Specifically, the FBI has jurisdiction to investigate felony killings of state law enforcement officers (28 U.S.C. § 540), violent crimes against interstate travelers

(28 U.S.C. § 540A), and serial killers (28 U.S.C. § 540B). Authority to investigate these matters is contingent on receiving a request by an appropriate state official.

B. (U) **Threats to the National Security**

(U) The FBI has authority to investigate threats to the national security pursuant to executive orders, Attorney General authorities, and various statutory sources. (See E.O. 12333; 50 U.S.C. §§ 401 et seq.; 50 U.S.C. §§ 1801 et seq.)

(U) "Threats to the national security" are specifically defined to mean: international terrorism; espionage and other intelligence activities, sabotage, and assassination, conducted by, for, or on behalf of foreign powers, organizations, or persons; foreign computer intrusion; and other matters determined by the Attorney General, consistent with Executive Order 12333 or any successor order. (AGG-Dom, Part VII.S)

C. (U) **Foreign Intelligence Collection**

(U) The FBI authority to collect foreign intelligence derives from a mixture of administrative and statutory sources. (See E.O. 12333; 50 U.S.C. §§ 401 et seq.; 50 U.S.C. §§ 1801 et seq.; 28 U.S.C. § 532 note (incorporates the Intelligence Reform and Terrorism Protection Act, P.L. 108-458 §§ 2001-2003).

(U) "Foreign Intelligence" is defined as information relating to the capabilities, intentions, or activities of foreign governments or elements thereof, foreign organizations or foreign persons, or international terrorists. (AGG-Dom, Part VII.E)

7.5. (U) Predication

(U) A full investigation may be initiated if there is an "articulable factual basis" that reasonably indicates one of the following circumstances exists:

A. (U) An activity constituting a federal crime or a threat to the national security has or may have occurred, is or may be occurring, or will or may occur and the investigation may obtain information relating to the activity or the involvement or role of an individual, group, or organization in such activity.

B. (U) An individual, group, organization, entity, information, property, or activity is or may be a target of attack, victimization, acquisition, infiltration, or recruitment in connection with criminal activity in violation of federal law or a threat to the national security and the investigation may obtain information that would help to protect against such activity or threat.

C. (U) The investigation may obtain foreign intelligence that is responsive to a Positive Foreign Intelligence Requirement, as defined in DIOG Section 7.4.C.

(U//FOUO)

   (i)   (U//FOUO)

   (ii)   (U//FOUO)

b2
b7E

(iii)   (U//FOUO)[   ]

b2
b7E

7.6. (U//FOUO) Standards for Initiating or Approving a Full Investigation

(U//FOUO) Before initiating or approving the conduct of a full investigation, an FBI employee or approving official must determine whether:

A. (U//FOUO) An authorized purpose and adequate predication exist for initiating a full investigation;

B. (U//FOUO) The full investigation is based on factors other than the exercise of First Amendment activities or the race, ethnicity, national origin or religion of the subject; and

C. (U//FOUO) The full investigation is an appropriate use of personnel and financial resources.

7.7. (U) Duration, Approval, Notice, Documentation and File Review

A. (U//FOUO) **Initiation:** The purpose of and predication for a full investigation must be documented in the initiating EC. The effective date of the full investigation is the date the final approval authority (e.g., SSA or SAC) approves the EC.

1. (U//FOUO) **By a Field Office:** The initiation of a full investigation for circumstances described in Sections 7.5.A and 7.5.B by a Field Office requires prior approval of the SSA with written notification to the appropriate FBIHQ substantive Unit. The initiation of a full investigation of a United States person relating to a threat to the national security for circumstances described in Sections 7.5.A and 7.5.B requires the approval of the Field Office SSA with written notification to the appropriate FBIHQ substantive Unit. The FBIHQ substantive Unit must notify DOJ NSD as soon as practicable but in all events within 30 calendar days after the initiation of the investigation.

2. (U//FOUO) **By FBIHQ:** The initiation of a full investigation for circumstances described in Sections 7.5.A and 7.5.B by FBIHQ requires prior approval of the Unit Chief with written notification to the appropriate Field Office. The initiation of a full investigation by FBIHQ of a United States person relating to a threat to the national security for circumstances described in Sections 7.5.A and 7.5.B requires the approval of the Unit Chief with written notification to the appropriate Field Office and notice to DOJ NSD as soon as practicable but in all events within 30 days after initiation of the investigation.

3. (U//FOUO) **Sensitive Investigative Matter:** The initiation of a full investigation involving a <u>sensitive investigative matter</u>:

    a. (U//FOUO) **By a Field Office:** requires CDC review, SAC approval, and written notification to the appropriate FBIHQ substantive Unit Chief and Section Chief. Additionally, the Field Office must notify, in writing, the United States Attorney, if required. The appropriate FBIHQ Section must notify, in writing, the DOJ Criminal Division or NSD as soon as practicable, but no later than 30 calendar days after the initiation of the investigation. The notice must identify all known sensitive investigative matters involved in the investigation (see classified appendix for additional notice requirements). If a sensitive investigative matter arises after the initiation of a full investigation, investigative activity must cease

88

until CDC review and SAC approval are acquired and notice is furnished as specified above.

    b. (U//FOUO) **By FBIHQ:** requires OGC review, Section Chief approval, and written notification to the United States Attorney and the appropriate Field Office or the DOJ Criminal Division or NSD as soon as practicable, but no later than 30 calendar days after the initiation of such an investigation. The notice must identify all known sensitive investigative matters involved in the investigation (see classified appendix for additional notice requirements). If a sensitive investigative matter arises after the initiation of a full investigation, investigative activity must cease until OGC review and Section Chief approval are acquired and notice is furnished as specified above. (AGG-Dom, Part II.B.5.a)

4. (U//FOUO) The initiation of a full investigation in order to collect positive foreign intelligence must be approved as provided in Section 9. Additionally, written notification to FBIHQ CMS and DOJ NSD is required as soon as practicable but no later than 30 calendar days after the initiation of the investigation.

5. (U//FOUO) The EAD for the National Security Branch must notify the Deputy Attorney General if FBI Headquarters disapproves a Field Office's initiation of a full investigation relating to a threat to the national security on the ground that the predication for the investigation is insufficient, and the EAD for the National Security Branch is responsible for establishing a system that will allow for the prompt retrieval of such denials. (AGG-Dom, Part II.B.5.d)

B. (U//FOUO) **Closing:** When closing the full investigation, the Field Office or FBIHQ will provide the reason for closing the investigation. When closing a full investigation, the SSA or Unit Chief must ensure that all pending investigative methods have been completed/ terminated (e.g., mail covers and pen register/trap and trace). Although there is no duration requirement for a full investigation, the investigation must be closed upon all investigative activity being exhausted.

1. (U//FOUO) Closing a full investigation initiated by a Field Office requires approval from the SSA. Notification to the substantive FBIHQ Unit may be required by program policy.

2. (U//FOUO) Closing a full investigation initiated by FBIHQ requires approval from the Unit Chief and notification to the appropriate Field Office.

3. (U//FOUO) Closing a full investigation initiated by a Field Office involving a sensitive investigative matter requires approval from the SAC and written notification to the FBIHQ substantive Unit and Section.

4. (U//FOUO) Closing a full investigation initiated by FBIHQ involving a sensitive investigative matter requires approval from the Section Chief and written notification to the appropriate Field Office.

5. (U//FOUO) Closing a full investigation for the purpose of positive foreign intelligence collection requires the approval of FBIHQ CMS.

C. (U//FOUO) **File Review:** Supervisory file reviews must be conducted at least once every 90 days in accordance with Section 3.4. File reviews for probationary FBI employees must be conducted at least every 60 days.

D. (U//FOUO) **Annual Letterhead Memorandum:** Annual letterhead memoranda regarding the status of full investigations are not required by the AGG-Dom; however,

b2
b7E

7.8. (U//FOUO) Standards for Initiating or Approving the Use of an Authorized Investigative Method

(U//FOUO) Prior to initiating or approving the use of an investigative method, an FBI employee or approving official must determine whether:

A. (U//FOUO) The use of the particular investigative method is likely to further the purpose of the full investigation;

B. (U//FOUO) The investigative method selected is the least intrusive method, reasonable under the circumstances;

C. (U//FOUO) If the full investigation is for collecting positive foreign intelligence, the FBI must operate openly and consensually with a United States person, to the extent practicable; and

D. (U//FOUO) The method to be used is an appropriate use of personnel and financial resources.

7.9. (U) Authorized Investigative Methods in Full Investigations

(U) All lawful methods may be used in a full investigation, unless the investigation is to collect foreign intelligence. The use or dissemination of information obtained by the use of these methods must comply with the AGG-Dom and DIOG Section 14. See foreign intelligence collection Section 9 for more information regarding use of authorized investigative methods.

A. (U) Obtain publicly available information.

B. (U) Access and examine FBI and other DOJ records, and obtain information from any FBI or other DOJ personnel.

C. (U) Access and examine records maintained by, and request information from, other federal, state, local, or tribal, or foreign governmental entities or agencies.

D. (U) Use online services and resources (whether non-profit or commercial).

E. (U) Use and recruit human sources in conformity with the AGG-CHS.

F. (U) Interview or request information from members of the public and private entities.

G. (U) Accept information voluntarily provided by governmental or private entities.

H. (U) Engage in observation or surveillance not requiring a court order.

I. (U) Grand Jury Subpoenas for telephone or electronic mail subscriber information (see also 'P' below).

J. (U) Mail covers. (AGG-Dom, Part V.A.2)

K. (U) Physical searches of personal or real property where a warrant or court order is not legally required because there is no reasonable expectation of privacy (e.g., trash covers). (AGG-Dom, Part V.A.3)

L. (U) Consensual monitoring of communications, including consensual computer monitoring, subject to legal review by the CDC or the FBI OGC. When a sensitive monitoring circumstance is involved, the monitoring must be approved by the DOJ Criminal Division or, if the investigation concerns a threat to the national security, by the DOJ NSD. (AGG-Dom, Part V.A.4)

(U) Sensitive monitoring circumstances include:

1. (U) Investigation of a member of Congress, a federal judge, a member of the Executive Branch at Executive Level IV or above, or a person who has served in such capacity within the previous two years (Executive Level I through IV are defined in 5 U.S.C. §§ 5312-5315);

2. (U) Investigation of the Governor, Lieutenant Governor, or Attorney General of any state or territory, or a judge or justice of the highest court of any state or territory, concerning an offense involving bribery, conflict of interest, or extortion related to the performance of official duties;

3. (U) A party to the communication is in the custody of the Bureau of Prisons or the United States Marshal Service or is being or has been afforded protection in the Witness Security Program; or

4. (U) The Attorney General, the Deputy Attorney General, or an Assistant Attorney General has requested that the FBI obtain prior approval for the use of consensual monitoring in a specific investigation. (AGG-Dom, Part VII.A and O)

(U//FOUO) **Note:** See classified appendix for additional information.

(U//FOUO) **Note:** For those state, local and tribal governments that do not sanction or provide a law enforcement exception available to the FBI for one-party consensual recording of communications with persons within their jurisdiction, the SAC must approve the consensual monitoring of communications as an OIA, as discussed in Section 17. Prior to the SAC authorizing the OIA, one-party consent must be acquired. The SAC may delegate this OIA approval authority to an ASAC or SSA.

M. (U) Use of closed-circuit television, direction finders, and other monitoring devices, subject to legal review by the CDC or the FBI OGC. (The methods described in this paragraph usually do not require a court order or warrant unless they involve an intrusion into an area where there is a reasonable expectation of privacy or non-consensual monitoring of communications, but legal review is necessary to ensure compliance with all applicable legal requirements.) (AGG-Dom, Part V.A.5)

N. (U) Polygraph examinations. (AGG-Dom, Part V.A.6)

O. (U) Undercover operations. In investigations relating to activities in violation of federal criminal law that do not concern threats to the national security or foreign intelligence, undercover operations must be carried out in conformity with *The Attorney General's Guidelines on Federal Bureau of Investigation Undercover Operations*. Investigations that are not subject to the preceding sentence because they concern threats to the national security or foreign intelligence undercover operations involving religious or political organizations must be reviewed and approved by FBI Headquarters, with participation by the DOJ NSD in the review process. (AGG-Dom, Part V.A.7)

P. (U) Compulsory process as authorized by law, including grand jury subpoenas and other subpoenas, National Security Letters (15 U.S.C. §§ 1681u, 1681v; 18 U.S.C. § 2709; 12 U.S.C. § 3414[a][5][A]; 50 U.S.C. § 436), and FISA orders for the production of tangible things. (50 U.S.C. §§ 1861-63). (AGG-Dom, Part V.A.8)

Q. (U) Accessing stored wire and electronic communications and transactional records in conformity with chapter 121 of title 18, United States Code (18 U.S.C. §§ 2701-2712). (AGG-Dom, Part V.A.9)

R. (U) Use of pen registers and trap and trace devices in conformity with chapter 206 of title 18, United States Code (18 U.S.C. §§ 3121-3127) or FISA (50 U.S.C. §§ 1841-1846). (AGG-Dom, Part V.A.10)

(U) **The following investigative methods can only be used in full investigations:**

S. (U) Electronic surveillance in conformity with chapter 119 of Title 18, United States Code (18 U.S.C. §§ 2510-2522), FISA, or Executive Order 12333 § 2.5. (AGG-Dom, Part V.A.11)

T. (U) Physical searches, including mail openings, in conformity with Rule 41 of the Federal Rules of Criminal Procedure, FISA, or Executive Order 12333 § 2.5. The classified appendix to the DIOG, Appendix G, provides additional information regarding certain searches. (AGG-Dom, Part V.A.12)

U. (U) Acquisition of foreign intelligence information in conformity with Title VII of FISA. (AGG-Dom, Part V.A.13)

7.10. (U) Sensitive Investigative Matter / Academic Nexus / Buckley Amendment

(U//FOUO) The title/case caption of the opening or subsequent EC for a full investigation involving a sensitive investigative matter must contain the words "Sensitive Investigative Matter." DIOG Section 10 contains the required approval authority and factors to be considered when determining whether to conduct or to approve a predicated investigation involving a sensitive investigative matter. The AGG-Dom defines sensitive investigative matter as follows:

A. (U//FOUO) **Sensitive Investigative Matter:** An investigative matter involving the activities of a domestic public official or political candidate (involving corruption or a threat to the national security), religious or political organization or individual prominent in such an organization, or news media, or any other matter which, in the judgment of the official authorizing an investigation, should be brought to the attention of FBI Headquarters and other DOJ officials. (AGG-Dom, Part VII.N). As a matter of FBI policy, "judgment" means that the decision of the authorizing official is discretionary. DIOG Section 10 and/or the DIOG classified Appendix G define domestic public official, political candidate, religious or political organization or individual prominent in such an organization, and news media.

B. (U//FOUO) **Academic Nexus:**

b2
b7E

> [redacted]

(U//FOUO) The sensitivity related to an academic institution arises from the American tradition of "academic freedom" (e.g., an atmosphere in which students and faculty are free to express unorthodox ideas and views and to challenge conventional thought without fear of repercussion). Academic freedom does not mean, however, that academic institutions are off limits to FBI investigators in pursuit of information or individuals of legitimate investigative interest.

b2
b7E

(U//FOUO) For matters not considered a sensitive investigative matter [redacted] see the DIOG classified Appendix G.

C. (U//FOUO) **Buckley Amendment:** Although not a sensitive investigative matter, a request for "academic records" must only be made pursuant to the provisions of the Buckley Amendment (The Family Educational Rights and Privacy Act of 1974, 20 U.S.C. § 1232[g], as amended by Public Law 107-56 ["USA PATRIOT Act"]). An FBI employee is prohibited from receiving "academic records" that have not been properly requested pursuant to the Buckley Amendment. The definition of "academic records" is very broad and covers almost all records about a student other than public, student directory-type information published by the institution. The Buckley Amendment contains a penalty provision for those institutions that improperly provide academic records to law enforcement agencies. [redacted]

b2
b7E

> [redacted]

(U//FOUO) A Buckley Amendment request for academic records cannot be made during an assessment. In a predicated investigation, a request for academic records must be made pursuant to the Buckley Amendment.

7.11. (U) Program Specific Investigative Requirements

(U//FOUO) Because of the many investigative programs within the FBI, a single universal requirement will not adequately address every program. To facilitate compliance within an existing program, the FBI employee should consult the relevant program policy guidance.

8.   (U) Enterprise Investigations

8.1. (U) Overview

(U) Enterprise investigations may only be opened and operated as full investigations and are subject to the same requirements that apply to full investigations described in Section 7. Enterprise investigations focus on groups or organizations that may be involved in the most serious criminal or national security threats to the public, as described in Section 8.5 below. Enterprise investigations cannot be conducted as preliminary investigations or assessments, nor may they be conducted for the sole purpose of collecting positive foreign intelligence. See Section 8.2, below, regarding preliminary investigations and assessments.

8.2. (U) Purpose, Scope and Definitions

(U) The term "enterprise" includes any partnership, corporation, association, or other legal entity, and any union or group of individuals associated in fact, although not a legal entity. The purpose of an enterprise investigation is to examine the structure, scope, and nature of the group or organization including: its relationship, if any, to a foreign power; the identity and relationship of its members, employees, or other persons who may be acting in furtherance of its objectives; its finances and resources; its geographical dimensions; its past and future activities and goals; and its capacity for harm. (AGG-Dom, Part II.C.2)

(U//FOUO) Although an enterprise investigation may not be conducted as a preliminary investigation, a preliminary investigation may be used to determine whether a group or organization is a criminal or terrorist enterprise if the FBI has "information or an allegation" that an activity constituting a federal crime or a threat to the national security has or may have occurred, is or may be occurring, or will or may occur, and the investigation may obtain information relating to the activity of the group or organization in such activity. An assessment may also be initiated to determine whether a group or organization is involved in activities constituting violations of federal criminal law or threats to the national security.

8.3. (U) Civil Liberties and Privacy

(U) The pursuit of legitimate investigative goals without infringing upon the exercise of constitutional freedoms is a challenge that the FBI meets through the application of sound judgment and discretion. In order to further ensure that civil liberties are not undermined by the conduct of criminal and national security investigations, every full investigation, including an enterprise investigation under this subsection, must have an identified authorized purpose and adequate predication.

(U) No investigative activity, including enterprise investigations, may be taken solely on the basis of activities that are protected by the First Amendment or on the race, ethnicity, national origin or religion of the subject. Enterprise investigations of groups and organizations must focus on activities related to the threats or crimes being investigated, not solely on First Amendment activities or on the race, ethnicity, national origin or religion of the members of the group or organization. In this context, it is particularly important clearly to identify and document the law enforcement or national security basis of the enterprise investigation.

> (U//FOUO) **Example:** Groups who communicate with each other or with members of the public in any form in pursuit of social or political causes—

such as opposing war or foreign policy, protesting government actions, promoting certain religious beliefs, championing particular local, national, or international causes, or a change in government through non-criminal means, and actively recruit others to join their causes—have a fundamental constitutional right to do so. An enterprise investigation may not be initiated based solely on the exercise of these First Amendment rights.

(U) The AGG-Dom authorize all lawful investigative methods in the conduct of an enterprise investigation. Considering the effect on the privacy and civil liberties of individuals and the potential to damage the reputation of individuals, some of these investigative methods are more intrusive than others. The least intrusive method feasible is to be used, but the FBI must not hesitate to use any lawful method consistent with the AGG-Dom. A more intrusive method may be warranted in light of the seriousness of a criminal or national security threat.

(U) By emphasizing the use of the least intrusive means to obtain intelligence and/or evidence, FBI employees can effectively execute their duties while mitigating the potential negative impact on the privacy and civil liberties of all people encompassed within the investigation, including targets, witnesses, and victims. This principle is not intended to discourage FBI employees from seeking relevant and necessary intelligence, information, or evidence, but rather is intended to encourage FBI employees to choose the least intrusive—but still effective means—from the available options to obtain the material.

8.4. (U) Legal Authority

(U) A full investigation of a group or organization may be initiated as an enterprise investigation if there is an articulable factual basis for the investigation that reasonably indicates the group or organization may have engaged, or may be engaged in, or may have or may be engaged in planning or preparation or provision of support for: (AGG-Dom, Part II.C.1)

A. (U) A pattern of racketeering activity as defined in 18 U.S.C. § 1961(5);

B. (U) International terrorism, as defined in the AGG-Dom, Part VII.J. or other threat to the national security;

C. (U) Domestic terrorism as defined in 18 U.S.C. § 2331(5) involving a violation of federal criminal law;

D. (U) Furthering political or social goals wholly or in part through activities that involve force or violence and a violation of federal criminal law; or

E. (U) An offense described in 18 U.S.C. § 2332b(g)(5)(B) or 18 U.S.C. § 43.

8.5. (U) Predication

(U) An enterprise investigation is predicated when there is an articulable factual basis for the investigation that reasonably indicates the group or organization may have engaged or may be engaged in, or may have or may be engaged in, planning or preparation or provision of support for the matters identified in Section 8.4, above.

(U) The "articulable factual basis" for opening an enterprise investigation is met with the identification of a group whose statements made in furtherance of its objectives, or its conduct, demonstrate a purpose of committing crimes or securing the commission of crimes by others. The group's activities and statements of its members may be considered in combination to comprise the "articulable factual basis," even if the statements alone or activities alone would not warrant such a determination.

> (U//FOUO) **Examples** of situations in which an enterprise investigation may be opened:
>
> i. (U//FOUO)
>
> ii. (U//FOUO)   b2
>   b7E
>
> iii. (U//FOUO)

8.6. (U) Duration, Approval, Notice, Documentation and File Review

A. (U) Initiation:

1. (U//FOUO) **By a Field Office:** The initiation of an enterprise investigation by an FBI Field Office requires the prior approval of the Field Office SSA with written notification to the appropriate FBIHQ substantive Unit and DOJ (as discussed in greater detail below). FBIHQ Divisions may require specific facts to be included in this notification.   b2
    b7E

    Enterprise investigations involving sensitive investigative matters require CDC review, SAC approval, and written notification to the appropriate FBIHQ substantive Unit and DOJ.

    (U//FOUO) The responsible FBIHQ entity must notify the DOJ NSD or the Organized Crime and Racketeering Section (OCRS) of the initiation of an enterprise investigation, by a Field Office or by FBIHQ, as soon as practicable but no later than 30 days after the initiation of the investigation. The FBI Field Office must also notify any relevant USAO, except in counterintelligence investigations. See the DOJ NSD policy that governs notification to the USAO for counterintelligence investigations.

2. (U//FOUO) **By FBIHQ:** The initiation of an enterprise investigation by an FBIHQ Division requires the prior approval of the appropriate Section Chief with written notification to the appropriate Field Offices and DOJ (as discussed in greater detail below). Enterprise investigations involving sensitive investigative matters require OGC review, appropriate Assistant Director approval, and written notification to DOJ.

    (U//FOUO) The responsible FBIHQ entity must provide notification of an enterprise investigation initiation to the appropriate DOJ component (NSD or OCRS) as soon as practicable, but no later than 30 days after the initiation of the investigation. FBIHQ must notify any relevant USAO of the initiation of all enterprise investigations, except in counterintelligence investigations.

(U//FOUO) **Note:** For enterprise investigations that involve allegations that pertain to national security matters, the responsible DOJ component for the purpose of notification and reports is the NSD. For enterprise investigations relating to a pattern of racketeering activity that does not involve terrorism offenses, see 18 U.S.C. § 2332b(g)(5)(B), the responsible DOJ component is the Organized Crime and Racketeering Section of the Criminal Division. (AGG-Dom, Part II.C.3)

(U) The Assistant Attorney General for National Security or the Chief of the Organized Crime and Racketeering Section, as appropriate, may at any time request the FBI to provide a report on the status of an enterprise investigation and the FBI will provide such reports as requested. (AGG-Dom, Part II C.3.d)

B. (U//FOUO) **Closing:** When closing the enterprise investigation, the Field Office or FBIHQ will provide the reason for closing the investigation. When closing an enterprise investigation, the SSA or Unit Chief must ensure that all pending investigative methods have been completed/terminated (e.g., mail covers and pen register/trap and trace). Although there is no duration requirement for an enterprise investigation, the investigation must be closed upon all investigative activity being exhausted.

1. (U//FOUO) Closing an enterprise investigation initiated by a Field Office requires approval from the SSA with written notification to the appropriate FBIHQ substantive Unit. Unless advised contrary by the FBIHQ (UACB) substantive desk, the enterprise investigation can be closed 30 days after the date of notification to FBIHQ.

2. (U//FOUO) Closing an enterprise investigation initiated by FBIHQ requires approval from the Unit Chief and notification to the appropriate Field Office.

3. (U//FOUO) Closing an enterprise investigation initiated by a Field Office involving a sensitive investigative matter requires approval from the SAC, with written notification to the appropriate FBIHQ substantive Unit. The enterprise investigation can be closed 30 days after the notification to FBIHQ, UACB.

4. (U//FOUO) Closing an enterprise investigation initiated by FBIHQ involving a sensitive investigative matter requires approval from the Section Chief, and written notification to the appropriate Field Office.

C. (U//FOUO) **File Review:**

(U//FOUO) Supervisory file reviews must be conducted at least once every 90 days in accordance with Section 3.4. File reviews for probationary agents must be conducted at least once every 60 days.

9. (U) Foreign Intelligence

9.1. (U) Overview.

(U) Foreign intelligence is "information relating to the capabilities, intentions, or activities of foreign governments or elements thereof, foreign organizations, or foreign persons, or international terrorists." A "Foreign Intelligence Requirement" is a collection requirement issued under the authority of the DNI and accepted by the FBI DI. Additionally, the President, a USIC office designated by the President, the Attorney General, Deputy Attorney General, or other designated DOJ official may levy a Foreign Intelligence Requirement on the FBI. Foreign intelligence collection by the FBI is based upon requirements.

(U//FOUO) Foreign Intelligence Requirements issued by one of the parties listed above and accepted by the FBI DI will fall into one of two categories: (i) those that address national security issues that are within the FBI's core national security mission; and (ii) information relating to the capabilities, intentions, or activities of foreign governments or elements thereof, foreign organizations, foreign persons, or international terrorists which are not within the FBI's core national security mission.

(U//FOUO) Requirements which fall into the first category may correspond to FBI National Collection Requirements as defined in Section 5.11. FBI National Collection Requirements will only be addressed in properly authorized assessments or incidental to predicated investigations. (See the DI PG for specific requirements.)

(U//FOUO) Requirements which fall into the second category are known as Positive Foreign Intelligence Requirements and may only be addressed under the authorities described in this section. Assessments and full investigations intended to result in the collection of positive foreign intelligence must be based upon established requirements and approved by FBIHQ DI. Preliminary investigations for the sole purpose of collecting positive foreign intelligence are not authorized. Assessments and full investigations initiated for the purpose of positive foreign intelligence collection must be opened by FBIHQ CMS. For assessments, the authorized purpose and identified objective must be documented in the assessment file.

b2
b7E

(U//FOUO) "The general guidance of the FBI's foreign intelligence collection activities by DNI-authorized requirements does not limit the FBI's authority to conduct investigations supportable on the basis of its other authorities—to investigate federal crimes and threats to the national security—in areas in which the information sought also falls under the definition of foreign intelligence." (AGG-Dom, Introduction A.3) Accordingly, the AGG-Dom authorizes the collection of foreign intelligence incidental to predicated criminal, counterintelligence, counterterrorism, cyber, and weapons of mass destruction investigations.

(U//FOUO) FBI National Collection Requirements which address national security issues that are within the FBI's core national security mission will be worked under FBI substantive case classifications (e.g., 200, 105, 315) as assessments. An assessment cannot be opened solely based upon an FBI National Collection Requirement. An authorized purpose (national security or criminal threat) must exist and the objective of the assessment must be clearly articulated when opening an authorized assessment. The authorized purpose and identified objective for all assessments must be documented in the assessment file.

(U//FOUO) **Example:**

(i) (U//FOUO)

b2
b7E
b7A

(ii) (U//FOUO)

b2
b7E

(U//FOUO)

b2
b7E

(U//FOUO) **Note:** FBIHQ DI provides specific guidance in its policy implementation guide regarding FBI National Collection Requirements, FBI Field Office Collection Requirements, and Positive Foreign Intelligence Requirements.

9.2. (U) Purpose and Scope

(U//FOUO) As stated above, foreign intelligence is "information relating to the capabilities, intentions, or activities of foreign governments or elements thereof, foreign organizations, or foreign persons, or international terrorists." The collection of positive foreign intelligence extends the sphere of the FBI's information-gathering activities beyond federal crimes and threats to the national security and permits the FBI to seek information regarding a broader range of matters relating to foreign powers, organizations, or persons that may be of interest to the conduct of the United States' foreign affairs. (AGG-Dom, Introduction A.3)

9.3. (U) Civil Liberties and Privacy

(U) Because the authority to collect positive foreign intelligence enables the FBI to obtain information pertinent to the United States' conduct of its foreign affairs, even if that information is not related to criminal activity or threats to the national security, the information so gathered may concern lawful activities. Accordingly, the FBI must operate openly and consensually with a United States person to the extent practicable when collecting positive foreign intelligence. (AGG-Dom, Introduction A.3)

(U) The pursuit of legitimate investigative goals without infringing upon the exercise of constitutional freedoms is a challenge that the FBI meets through the application of sound judgment and discretion. In order to further ensure that civil liberties are not undermined, every assessment or full investigation involving the collection of positive foreign intelligence under this section must have an authorized purpose and an identified objective. Additionally, the authorized purpose and objective of any assessment conducted must be documented and retained as prescribed in Sections 5 and 14.

(U) No investigative activity, including the collection of positive foreign intelligence, may be taken solely on the basis of activities that are protected by the First Amendment or on the race, ethnicity, national origin or religion of the subject. Collection of positive foreign intelligence requires: (i) an assessment relating to a matter of foreign intelligence interest responsive to a Positive Foreign Intelligence Requirement; or (ii) a full investigation that is predicated on a Positive Foreign Intelligence Requirement.

(U) The AGG-Dom present investigators with a number of authorized investigative methods in the conduct of an assessment or full investigation to collect positive foreign intelligence. Considering the effect on the privacy and civil liberties of individuals and the potential to damage the reputation of individuals, some of these investigative methods are more intrusive than others. The least intrusive method feasible is to be used, but the FBI must not hesitate to use any lawful method consistent with the AGG-Dom. For further explanation of the least intrusive method refer to Section 4.

(U) Moreover, when collecting positive foreign intelligence either as part of an assessment related to a matter of foreign intelligence interest or as part of a full investigation predicated on a Positive Foreign Intelligence Requirement, the FBI must operate openly and consensually with a United States person, to the extent practicable.

(U) By emphasizing the use of the least intrusive means to collect positive foreign intelligence and by emphasizing the need to operate openly and consensually with a United States person, to the extent practicable, FBI employees can effectively execute their duties while mitigating the potential negative impact on the privacy and civil liberties of all people encountered as part of the collection. This principle is not intended to discourage FBI employees from seeking relevant and necessary positive foreign intelligence or evidence, but rather is intended to make sure FBI employees choose the least intrusive—but still effective—means from the available options to obtain the information.

9.4. (U) Legal Authority

(U) The FBI's legal authority to collect positive foreign intelligence derives from a mixture of administrative and statutory sources. (See E.O. 12333; 50 U.S.C. §§ 401 et seq.; 50 U.S.C. §§ 1801 et seq.; 28 U.S.C. § 532 note [incorporates the Intelligence Reform and Terrorism Protection Act, P.L. 108-458 §§ 2001-2003]). In collecting positive foreign intelligence, the FBI will be guided by Collection Requirements issued under the authority of the DNI, including the

National Intelligence Priorities Framework and the National HUMINT Collection Directives, or any successor directives issues under the authority of the DNI and accepted by FBIHQ DI.

A. (U) Assessment Activities

(U//FOUO) As discussed in Section 5 of the DIOG, the AGG-Dom authorize six types of assessments, one of which specifically applies to collection of positive foreign intelligence as follows: "seeking information, proactively or in response to investigative leads on matters of foreign intelligence interest responsive to foreign intelligence requirements." Positive Foreign Intelligence Requirements can be found on the DI's Collection Management Section website. Further instructions on the collection of positive foreign intelligence are contained in the DI PG.

B. (U) Full Investigation Activities

(U//FOUO) As discussed in Section 7 of the DIOG, the AGG-Dom cites three predication circumstances warranting a full investigation, one of which specifically applies to collection of positive foreign intelligence: "The full investigation may obtain foreign intelligence that is responsive to a foreign intelligence requirement."

(U//FOUO) Predicated positive foreign intelligence collection originates when the Office of the DNI levies a foreign intelligence collection requirement on the FBI and the DI accepts the requirement as one to which the FBI will endeavor to respond to as part of its Positive Foreign Intelligence Program.

(U//FOUO) A full investigation to collect positive foreign intelligence is appropriate only when a DNI-authorized requirement exists for a particular issue and that requirement has been accepted by FBIHQ DI.

9.5. (U//FOUO) Duration, Approval, Notice, Documentation, File Review and FBIHQ Standards for Approving the Initiation of Positive Foreign Intelligence Investigations

A. (U//FOUO) Positive Foreign Intelligence Collection Authorities

(U//FOUO) The FBIHQ CMS is responsible for promulgating FBI policy and oversight of the Foreign Intelligence Collection Program (FICP). FBIHQ CMS will provide notice to the DOJ NSD upon the initiation of a positive foreign intelligence investigation. To ensure that all positive foreign intelligence collection is focused on authorized Positive Foreign Intelligence Requirements, only FBIHQ CMS may approve the initiation of a positive foreign intelligence assessment or full investigation[   ] or as otherwise determined by DI). [   ] Field offices must request, by EC, FBIHQ CMS approval to open such assessments and full investigations.

b2
b7E

B. (U//FOUO) Standards to be Considered When Initiating an Assessment or Full Foreign Intelligence Investigation to Collect Positive Foreign Intelligence

(U//FOUO) Before initiating or approving an assessment or full investigation for the purpose of collecting positive foreign intelligence, the approving official must determine whether:

1. (U//FOUO) An authorized purpose and objective exists for the conduct of the assessment or an authorized purpose and adequate predication exists for initiating a full investigation;

2. (U//FOUO) The assessment or full investigation is not based solely on the exercise of First Amendment activities or on the race, ethnicity, national origin or religion of the subject; and

3. (U//FOUO) The assessment or full investigation is an appropriate use of personnel and financial resources.

9.6. (U//FOUO) Standards for Initiating or Approving the Use of an Authorized Investigative Method

(U//FOUO) Before initiating or approving the use of an investigative method in an assessment or full investigation for the purpose of collecting positive foreign intelligence, an FBI employee or approving official must determine whether:

A. (U//FOUO) The use of the particular investigative method is likely to further the purpose of the assessment or full investigation;

B. (U//FOUO) The investigative method selected is the least intrusive method, reasonable under the circumstances and, if taken relative to a United States person, the method involves open and consensual activities, to the extent practicable;

C. (U//FOUO) If open and consensual activity would likely be successful, then covert non-consensual contact with a United States person may not be approved.

D. (U//FOUO) In the case of an assessment, the anticipated value of the assessment justifies the use of the selected investigative method or methods; and

E. (U//FOUO) The investigative method is an appropriate use of personnel and financial resources.

9.7. (U) Authorized Investigative Methods in Foreign Intelligence Assessments and Predicated Investigations

(U//FOUO) Prior to initiating or approving the use of a method, an FBI employee and approving official will apply the standards as provided in Section 9.6. With the exceptions noted below, all lawful assessment methods may be used during positive foreign intelligence assessments. With the exceptions noted below, all lawful methods may be used during a full investigation to collect positive foreign intelligence. **If actions are to be taken with respect to a United States person, the method used must include open and consensual activities, to the extent practicable.**

A. (U) **Assessments** (see DIOG Section 5.9 for a complete description of the following methods that may be used in assessments):

1. (U) Obtain publicly available information.

2. (U) Engage in observation or surveillance not requiring a court order.

3. (U) Access and examine FBI and other DOJ records, and obtain information from any FBI or other DOJ personnel.

4. (U) Access and examine records maintained by, and request information from, other federal, state, local, or tribal, or foreign governmental entities or agencies.

5. (U) Use online services and resources (whether non-profit or commercial).

6. (U) Interview or request information from members of the public and private entities.

7. (U) Accept information voluntarily provided by governmental or private entities.

8. (U) Use and recruit human sources in conformity with the AGG-CHS.

(U//FOUO) **Note:** The use of Federal Grand Jury Subpoenas, to include subpoenas for telephone or electronic mail subscriber information, is not authorized in a positive foreign intelligence assessment.

B. (U) **Full Investigations:**

(U) In addition to the authorized methods listed in Section 9.7.A, above, the following lawful methods may also be used in full investigations opened for the purpose of collecting positive foreign intelligence:

1. (U) Physical searches of personal or real property where a warrant or court order is not legally required because there is no reasonable expectation of privacy (e.g., trash covers). (AGG-Dom, Part V.A.3)

2. (U) Consensual monitoring of communications, including consensual computer monitoring, subject to legal review by the CDC or the FBI OGC. Where a sensitive monitoring circumstance is involved, the monitoring must be approved by the DOJ Criminal Division or, if the investigation concerns a threat to the national security, by the DOJ NSD. (AGG-Dom, Part V.A.4)

   (U//FOUO) **Note:** See the classified appendix for additional information.

   (U//FOUO) **Note:** For those state, local and tribal governments that do not sanction or provide a law enforcement exception available to the FBI for one-party consent recording of communications with persons within their jurisdiction, the SAC must approve the consensual monitoring of communications as an OIA. Prior to the SAC authorizing the OIA, one-party consent must be acquired. The SAC may delegate the OIA approval authority to an ASAC or SSA.

3. (U) Use of closed-circuit television, direction finders, and other monitoring devices, subject to legal review by the CDC or the FBI OGC. (The methods described in this paragraph usually do not require court orders or warrants unless they involve an intrusion into an area where there is a reasonable expectation of privacy or non-consensual monitoring of communications, but legal review is necessary to ensure compliance with all applicable legal requirements.) (AGG-Dom, Part V.A.5)

4. (U) Polygraph examinations (AGG-Dom, Part V.A.6)

5. (U) Undercover operations. Undercover operations involving religious or political organizations conducted for the purpose of collecting positive foreign intelligence must be reviewed and approved by FBIHQ, with participation by the DOJ NSD in the review process. (AGG-Dom, Part V.A.7)

6. (U//FOUO) Use of pen registers and trap and trace devices in conformity with FISA (50 U.S.C. §§ 1841-1846), for non-United States persons only. (AGG-Dom, Part V.A.10)

7. (U) Electronic surveillance in conformity with FISA or E.O. 12333 § 2.5. (AGG-Dom, Part V.A.11)

8. (U//FOUO) Physical searches, including mail openings, in conformity with FISA or E.O. 12333 § 2.5. The classified appendix to the DIOG provides additional information regarding certain searches. (AGG-Dom, Part V.A.12)

9. (U) Acquisition of positive foreign intelligence information in conformity with Title VII of FISA. (AGG-Dom, Part V.A.13)

10. (U//FOUO) Obtaining a business records order pursuant to FISA, 50 U.S.C. §§ 1861-83, for records relating to a non-United States person only.

9.8. (U//FOUO) Investigative Methods Not Authorized During Foreign Intelligence Investigations

(U//FOUO) The following investigative methods are not permitted for the purpose of collecting positive foreign intelligence:

A. (U//FOUO) National Security Letters (15 U.S.C. §§ 1681u, 1681v; 18 U.S.C. § 2709; 12 U.S.C. § 341[a][5][A]; 50 U.S.C. § 436);

B. (U//FOUO) Obtaining a business records order pursuant to FISA, 50 U.S.C. §§ 1861-1863, for records relating to a United States person;

C. (U//FOUO) Use of pen registers and trap and trace devices in conformity with FISA (50 U.S.C. §§ 1841-1846) on a United States person;

D. (U//FOUO) Use of pen registers and trap and trace devices in conformity with chapter 206 of 18 U.S.C. §§ 3121-3127;

E. (U//FOUO) Mail covers;

F. (U//FOUO) Compulsory process as authorized by law, including grand jury subpoenas and other subpoenas (e.g., Administrative Subpoena); and

G. (U//FOUO) Accessing stored wire and electronic communications and transactional records in conformity with chapter 121 of title 18, United States Code (18 U.S.C. §§ 2701-2712). (AGG-Dom, Part V.A.9)

9.9. (U) Sensitive Investigative Matter

(U//FOUO) The title/case caption of the opening or subsequent EC for a positive foreign intelligence assessment involving a sensitive investigative matter must contain the words "Assessment" and "Sensitive Investigative Matter." The title/case caption of the opening or subsequent EC for a full investigation for the collection of positive foreign intelligence involving a sensitive investigative matter must contain the words "Sensitive Investigative Matter." DIOG Section 10 contains the required approval authorities and factors to be considered relative to an assessment or a predicated investigation involving a sensitive investigative matter. The AGG-Dom defines sensitive investigative matter as follows:

A. (U//FOUO) **Sensitive Investigative Matter:** An investigative matter involving the activities of a domestic public official or political candidate (involving corruption or a threat to the national security), religious or political organization or individual prominent in such an organization, or news media, or any other matter which, in the judgment of the official authorizing an investigation, should be brought to the attention of FBI Headquarters and other DOJ officials. (AGG-Dom, Part VII.N.) As a matter of FBI policy, "judgment" means that the decision of the authorizing official is discretionary. DIOG Section 10 and/or the DIOG classified Appendix G define domestic public official, political candidate, religious or political organization or individual prominent in such an organization, and news media.

All positive foreign intelligence assessments or full investigations involving a sensitive investigative matter must be reviewed by the CDC, approved by the SAC, and approved by the appropriate FBIHQ DI Section Chief. (see DIOG Section 9.10 below)

B. (U//FOUO) **Academic Nexus:**

b2
b7E

(U//FOUO) The sensitivity related to an academic institution arises from the American tradition of "academic freedom" (e.g., an atmosphere in which students and faculty are free to express unorthodox ideas and views and to challenge conventional thought without fear of repercussion). Academic freedom does not mean, however, that academic institutions are off limits to FBI investigators in pursuit of information or individuals of legitimate investigative interest.

(U//FOUO) [   ] see the DIOG classified Appendix G.

9.10. (U) Approval and Notification

A. (U) **Initiation**

(U//FOUO) The authorized purpose of an assessment or full investigation must be documented in the initiating EC.

1. (U//FOUO) **Approval to Initiate an Assessment to Collect Positive Foreign Intelligence:** No assessment for the purpose of seeking information relating to matters of positive foreign intelligence interest responsive to a Positive Foreign Intelligence Requirement may be initiated without prior approval from FBIHQ CMS. After obtaining FBIHQ CMS approval [   ] The title/case caption of the opening EC must contain the word "Assessment," and the synopsis must identify the authorized purpose and the objective of the assessment.

b2
b7E

2. (U//FOUO) **Approval to Initiate a Full Investigation:** FBIHQ CMS will direct the initiation of full investigations based on Positive Foreign Intelligence Requirements.

3. (U//FOUO) **Approval to Initiate an Assessment or Full Investigation Involving a Sensitive Investigative Matter:** The initiation of either an assessment or full investigation to collect positive foreign intelligence involving a sensitive investigative matter must have prior CDC review, SAC approval and the appropriate FBIHQ DI Section Chief approval.

B. (U) **Notice**

1. (U//FOUO) Notification to DOJ is not required when an assessment to collect information relating to a matter of foreign intelligence interest responsive to a positive foreign intelligence requirement is initiated.

2. (U//FOUO) Notification to DOJ is required when a full investigation to collect information responsive to a foreign intelligence requirement is initiated. Notice must be forwarded from FBIHQ CMS to the DOJ NSD as soon as practicable but no later than 30 calendar days after the initiation of the investigation. (AGG-Dom, Part II.B.5)

C. (U) **Duration**

(U//FOUO) A foreign intelligence assessment and full investigation may continue for as long as necessary to achieve its purpose and objective if an assessment, or until the requirement is met in a full investigation.

D. (U) **File Review**

1. (U//FOUO) **Assessments:** Foreign intelligence assessments require recurring 90 day file reviews of the assessment file and any sub-file by the SSA/SIA. File reviews for probationary agents must be conducted at least every 60-days. The file review must:

    a. (U//FOUO) Evaluate the progress made toward the achievement of the authorized purpose and objective;

    b. (U//FOUO) Determine whether it is reasonably likely that information may be obtained that is relevant to the authorized objective, thereby warranting a continuation of the assessment;

    c. (U//FOUO) Determine whether the Field Office has appropriate access and ability to collect positive foreign intelligence in response to a requirement that has been accepted by FBIHQ DI; and

    d. (U//FOUO) Determine whether the assessment should be terminated.

2. (U//FOUO) **Full Investigations:** Supervisory file reviews must be conducted at least every 90 days in accordance with Section 3.4. File reviews for probationary agents must be conducted at least every 60-days.

E. (U) **Closing**

(U//FOUO) Upon its determination or at the request of the Field Office, only FBIHQ CMS may close an assessment or full investigation.

F. (U) **Annual Letterhead Memorandum**

1. (U//FOUO) **Field Office Responsibility:** All FIGs must submit an annual report on each positive foreign intelligence full investigation that was open for any period of time during the past calendar year. This report is due to FBIHQ CMS no later than January 30th of the calendar year following each year during which a full investigation is open and must consist of the following:

    a. (U//FOUO) The Positive Foreign Intelligence Requirement to which the investigation was responding;

b. (U//FOUO) All methods of collection used;

c. (U//FOUO) All sensitive matters encountered;

d. (U//FOUO) A list of all IIRs by number issued based on information collected during the investigation;

e. (U//FOUO) A summary of the positive foreign intelligence collected; and

f. (U//FOUO) The date the full investigation was opened and, if applicable, the date closed.

(U//FOUO) These reports should be submitted by electronic communication. The EC must be uploaded into ACS in a file number and in the applicable Foreign Intelligence Collection Program (FICP) case files as designated in the DI PG.

2. (U//FOUO) **FBIHQ Responsibility:** FBIHQ CMS must compile data from each Field Office regarding the scope and nature of the prior year's positive foreign intelligence collection program. The FBIHQ CMS must submit an annual comprehensive report of all activity described above to DOJ NSD no later than April 1st of each year. The report must include the following information:

a. (U//FOUO) The Positive Foreign Intelligence Requirement to which the investigation was responding;

b. (U//FOUO) All sensitive matters; and

c. (U//FOUO) The date the full investigation was opened and closed (if applicable).

9.11. (U) Retention of Information

(U//FOUO) FBIHQ CMS must maintain a database or records systems that permits the prompt retrieval of the status of each positive foreign intelligence collection full investigation (open or closed), the dates of opening and closing, and the basis for the full investigation.

10. (U) Sensitive Investigative Matter / Academic Nexus

10.1. (U) Overview

(U) Certain investigative matters should be brought to the attention of FBI management and DOJ officials because of the possibility of public notoriety and sensitivity. Accordingly, assessments and predicated investigations involving "sensitive investigative matters" have special approval and reporting requirements.

10.2. (U) Purpose, Scope and Definitions

(U//FOUO) A sensitive investigative matter is defined as an investigative matter involving the activities of a domestic public official or political candidate (involving corruption or a threat to the national security), religious or political organization or individual prominent in such an organization, or news media, or any other matter which, in the judgment of the official authorizing an investigation, should be brought to the attention of FBI Headquarters and other DOJ officials. (AGG-Dom, Part VII.N.) As a matter of FBI policy, "judgment" means that the decision of the authorizing official is discretionary. Descriptions for each of the officials and entities contained in the sensitive investigative matter definition are as follows:

A. (U//FOUO) **Domestic Public Official**—A domestic public official is an individual elected or appointed to a position of trust in a federal, state, local or tribal governmental entity or political subdivision thereof. A matter involving a domestic public official is a "sensitive investigative matter" if the assessment or predicated investigation involves corruption or a threat to the national security.

B. (U//FOUO) **Political candidate**—A political candidate is an individual who is seeking election to, or nomination for election to, or who has authorized others to explore on his or her behalf the possibility of election to, an office in a federal, state, local or tribal governmental entity or political subdivision thereof. As with domestic public officials, a matter involving a political candidate is a sensitive investigative matter if the assessment or predicated investigation involves corruption or a threat to the national security.

C. (U//FOUO) **Political organization or individual prominent in such an organization**—

D. (U//FOUO) **Religious organization or individual prominent in such an organization**—

b2
b7E

E. (U//FOUO) **Member of the media or a news organization—**

F. (U//FOUO) **Academic Nexus—**

b2
b7E

(U//FOUO) The sensitivity related to an academic institution arises from the American tradition of "academic freedom" (e.g., an atmosphere in which students and faculty are free to express unorthodox ideas and views and to challenge conventional thought without fear of repercussion). Academic freedom does not mean, however, that academic institutions are off limits to FBI investigators in pursuit of information or individuals of legitimate investigative interest.

(U//FOUO) [   ] see the classified appendix.

G. (U//FOUO) **Other Matters—**Any matter that in the judgment of the official authorizing an investigation that should be brought to the attention of FBIHQ and other Department of Justice officials. As a matter of FBI policy, "judgment" means that the decision of the authorizing official is discretionary.

10.3. (U//FOUO) Factors to Consider When Initiating or Approving an Investigative Activity Involving a Sensitive Investigative Matter

(U//FOUO) In addition to the standards for approving investigative activity in Sections 5, 6, 7 and 9, the following factors should be considered by the: (i) FBI employee who seeks to initiate an assessment or predicated investigation involving a sensitive investigative matter; (ii) CDC or OGC when reviewing such matters; and (iii) approving official in determining whether the assessment or predicated investigation involving a sensitive investigative matter should be authorized:

A. (U//FOUO) Seriousness/severity of the violation/threat;

B. (U//FOUO) Significance of the information sought to the violation/threat;

C. (U//FOUO) Probability that the proposed course of action will be successful;

D. (U//FOUO) Risk of public exposure, and if there is such a risk, the adverse impact or the perception of the adverse impact on civil liberties and public confidence; and

E. (U//FOUO) Risk to the national security or the public welfare if the proposed course of action is not approved (i.e., risk of doing nothing).

(U//FOUO) In the context of a sensitive investigative matter, particular care should be taken when considering whether the planned course of action is the least intrusive method feasible.

10.4. (U) Duration, Approval, Notice and Documentation

(U//FOUO) The following are required approval and notification levels for investigative activities involving sensitive investigative matters:

A. (U//FOUO) **Initiated by a Field Office:**

(U//FOUO) **Assessment:** An FBI employee may initiate assessment type one and two activities, as described in Section 5.6.A.1 and 2 (prompt checking of leads), without prior supervisory approval. However, because assessments involving sensitive investigative matters must be brought to the attention of FBI Field Office management, CDC review and SAC approval to continue the assessment must be acquired as soon as practicable. For assessment types 3, 4 and 6 assessments (see DIOG Section 5.6.A.3. 4 and 6) involving a sensitive investigative matter, prior CDC review and SAC approval is required. For assessment types 3, 4, and 6, as described in Section 5.6.A.3. 4 and 6, if a sensitive investigative matter arises after the initiation of an assessment, investigative activity must cease until CDC review and SAC approval is acquired.

(U//FOUO) Assessments involving a sensitive investigative matter do not require notification to DOJ or the United States Attorney. (AGG-Dom, Part II.B.5.a) All positive foreign intelligence collection assessments, regardless of whether they involve a sensitive investigative matter, require prior FBIHQ CMS approval. If a sensitive investigative matter arises after the initiation of a positive foreign intelligence collection assessment, notice must be provided to FBIHQ CMS.

(U//FOUO) **Predicated Investigation:** For all predicated investigations involving a sensitive investigative matter, prior CDC review and SAC approval is required, and the Field Office must provide written notification to the appropriate FBIHQ Unit Chief and Section Chief. Additionally, the Field Office must provide written notification to the United States Attorney or the appropriate FBIHQ Section must provide written notification to the DOJ Criminal Division or NSD, as soon as practicable, but no later than 30 calendar days after initiation of the predicated investigation. The notice must identify ⬚ ⬚ (see classified appendix for ⬚ ⬚

b2
b7E

(U//FOUO) If a sensitive investigative matter arises after the initiation of a predicated investigation, investigative activity must cease until CDC review and SAC approval is acquired and notice is furnished to the FBIHQ Unit and Section as specified above.

B. (U//FOUO) **Initiated by FBIHQ:**

(U//FOUO) **Assessment:** For assessment types 3, 4 and 6, as described in Section 5.6.A.3, 4 and 6, involving a sensitive investigative matter, OGC review and Section Chief approval is required. If a sensitive investigative matter arises after the initiation of an assessment, investigative activity must cease until OGC review and Section Chief approval is acquired.

(U//FOUO) Assessments involving a sensitive investigative matter do not require notification to DOJ or the United States Attorney. (AGG-Dom, Part II.B.5.a) All positive foreign intelligence collection assessments, regardless of whether they involve a sensitive investigative matter, require prior FBIHQ CMS approval. If a sensitive investigative matter arises after the initiation of a positive foreign intelligence collection assessment, notice must be provided to FBIHQ CMS.

(U//FOUO) **Predicated Investigation:** For predicated investigations involving a sensitive investigative matter, OGC review, Section Chief approval, and written notification to the United States Attorney, DOJ Criminal Division or DOJ NSD is required, as soon as practicable, but no later than 30 calendar days after the initiation of such an investigation. The notice must identify [   ] (see classified appendix [   ]

b2
b7E

(U//FOUO) If a sensitive investigative matter arises after the initiation of a predicated investigation, investigative activity must cease until OGC review and Section Chief approval is acquired and notice is furnished as specified above.

10.5. (U//FOUO) Distinction Between Sensitive Investigative Matter and Sensitive Circumstance

(U//FOUO) The term "sensitive investigative matter" should not be confused with the term "sensitive circumstance" as that term is used in undercover operations. A "sensitive circumstance" relates to an undercover operation requiring FBIHQ approval. A comprehensive list of sensitive circumstances for criminal activities is contained in the Attorney General's Guidelines on FBI Undercover Operations and in Section 11 of the DIOG for national security matters. The Criminal Undercover Operations Review Committee (CUORC) and [   ] must review and approve undercover operations that involve sensitive circumstances. The detailed policy for undercover operations is described in DIOG Section 11.8, the Field Guide for Undercover and Sensitive Operations (FGUSO), and the FBIHQ substantive Division program implementation guides.

b2
b7E

10.6. (U//FOUO) Sensitive Operations Review Committee

(U//FOUO) [   ]

b5

11. (U) Investigative Methods

11.1. (U) Overview

(U//FOUO) The conduct of assessments, predicated investigations and other activities authorized by the AGG-Dom may present choices between the use of different investigative methods (formerly investigative "techniques") that are each operationally sound and effective, but that are more or less intrusive, considering such factors as the effect on the privacy and civil liberties of individuals and the potential damage to reputation. The least intrusive method feasible is to be used in such situations. However, the choice of methods is a matter of judgment. The FBI is authorized to use any lawful method consistent with the AGG-Dom, even if intrusive, where the degree of intrusiveness is warranted in light of the seriousness of a criminal or national security threat or the strength of the information indicating its existence, or in light of the importance of foreign intelligence sought to the United States' interests. (AGG-Dom, Part I.C.2.)

(U) The availability of a particular investigative method in a particular case may depend upon the level of investigative activity (assessment, preliminary investigation, full investigation, assistance to other agencies).

11.1.1. (U) Least Intrusive Method

(U) The AGG-Dom requires that the "least intrusive" means or method be considered and—if operationally sound and effective—used to obtain intelligence or evidence in lieu of more intrusive methods. This principle is also reflected in Executive Order 12333, which governs the activities of the United States intelligence community. The concept of least intrusive method applies to the collection of intelligence and evidence.

(U) Selection of the least intrusive means is a balancing test as to which FBI employees must use common sense and sound judgment to effectively execute their duties while mitigating the potential negative impact on the privacy and civil liberties of all people encompassed within the assessment or predicated investigation, including targets, witnesses, and victims. This principle is not intended to discourage investigators from seeking relevant and necessary intelligence, information, or evidence, but rather is intended to encourage investigators to choose the least intrusive—yet still effective—means from the available options to obtain the material. Additionally, FBI employees should operate openly and consensually with United States persons to the extent practicable when collecting foreign intelligence that does not concern criminal activities or threats to the national security.

(U) Section 4.4 describes the least intrusive methods concept and the standards to be applied by FBI employees.

11.2. (U) Authorized Investigative Methods in Assessments and Predicated Investigations

(U) The below listed investigative methods may be used in assessments and predicated investigations. The use and/or dissemination of information obtained by the use of all authorized investigative methods must comply with the AGG-Dom and DIOG Section 14.

11.2.1. (U) Authorized Investigative Methods in Assessments

(AGG-Dom, Part II.A.4.)

(U//FOUO) An FBI employee must document on the FD-71, or in Guardian, the use of or the request and approval for the use of authorized investigative methods in type 1 and 2 assessments (see DIOG Section 5.6.A.1 and 2). By exception, certain assessment type 1 and 2 situations may require the use of an EC to document the use and approval of certain investigative methods. All authorized investigative methods in type 3, 4, and 6 assessments (see DIOG Section 5.6.A.3, 4 and 6) must use an EC to document the use of or the request and approval for the use of the applicable investigative method. For a detailed description of these methods see DIOG Section 5.9.

A. (U) Obtain publicly available information.

B. (U) Access and examine FBI and other Department of Justice records. and obtain information from any FBI or other Department of Justice personnel.

C. (U) Access and examine records maintained by. and request information from. other federal. state. local, or tribal. or foreign governmental entities or agencies.

D. (U) Use online services and resources (whether non-profit or commercial).

E. (U) Use and recruit human sources in conformity with the Attorney General's Guidelines Regarding the Use of FBI Confidential Human Sources.

F. (U) Interview or request information from members of the public and private entities.

G. (U) Accept information voluntarily provided by governmental or private entities.

H. (U) Engage in observation and conduct physical surveillance not requiring a court order.

I. (U//FOUO) Grand jury subpoenas for telephone or electronic mail subscriber information during type 1 and 2 assessments.

(U//FOUO) **Note:** In assessments, supervisory approval is required prior to use of the following investigative methods: certain interviews, tasking of a CHS, and physical surveillance not requiring a court order. During predicated investigations the supervisory approval requirements for these investigative methods may not apply.

11.2.2. (U) Authorized Investigative Methods in Preliminary Investigations

(AGG-Dom, Part V.A.1-10)

(U) In preliminary investigations the authorized methods include the following: [AGG-Dom, Part II.B. and Part V.A.]

A. (U) The investigative methods approved for assessments.

B. (U) Mail covers.

C. (U) Physical searches of personal or real property where a warrant or court order is not legally required because there is no reasonable expectation of privacy (e.g., trash covers).

D. (U) Consensual monitoring of communications, including consensual computer monitoring, subject to legal review by the CDC or the OGC. When a sensitive monitoring circumstance is involved, the monitoring must be approved by the DOJ Criminal Division or, if the investigation concerns a threat to the national security or foreign intelligence, by the DOJ National Security Division.

(U//FOUO) **Note:** For additional information, see the classified appendix.

(U//FOUO) **Note:** For those state, local and tribal governments that do not sanction or provide a law enforcement exception available to the FBI for one-party consent recording of communications with persons within their jurisdiction, the SAC must approve the consensual monitoring of communications as an OIA. Prior to the SAC authorizing the OIA, one-party consent must be acquired. The SAC may delegate the OIA approval authority to an ASAC or SSA.

E. (U) Use of closed-circuit television, direction finders, and other monitoring devices, subject to legal review by the CDC or the OGC. (The methods described in this paragraph usually do not require court orders or warrants unless they involve an intrusion into an area where there is a reasonable expectation of privacy or non-consensual monitoring of communications, but legal review is necessary to ensure compliance with all applicable legal requirements.)

F. (U) Polygraph examinations.

G. (U) Undercover operations. In investigations relating to activities in violation of federal criminal law that do not concern threats to the national security or foreign intelligence, undercover operations must be carried out in conformity with the Attorney General's Guidelines on Federal Bureau of Investigation Undercover Operations. In investigations that concern threats to the national security or foreign intelligence, undercover operations involving religious or political organizations must be reviewed and approved by FBI Headquarters, with participation by the DOJ National Security Division in the review process.

H. (U) Compulsory process as authorized by law, including grand jury subpoenas and other subpoenas, National Security Letters (15 U.S.C. §§ 1681u, 1681v; 18 U.S.C. § 2709; 12 U.S.C. § 3414[a][5][A]; 50 U.S.C. § 436, and FISA orders [50 U.S.C. §§ 1861-63]).

I. (U) Accessing stored wire and electronic communications and transactional records in conformity with chapter 121 of title 18, United States Code (18 U.S.C. §§ 2701-2712).

J. (U) Use of pen registers and trap and trace devices in conformity with chapter 206 of title 18, United States Code (18 U.S.C. §§ 3121-3127) or FISA (50 U.S.C. §§ 1841-1846).

11.2.3. **(U) Authorized Investigative Methods in Full Investigations**

(AGG-Dom, Part V.A.11-13)

(U) In full investigations, to include enterprise investigations, all investigative methods approved for assessments and preliminary investigations may be used. In addition, the three investigative methods listed below may only be used in full investigations:

A. (U) Electronic surveillance in conformity with chapter 119 of title 18, United States Code (18 U.S.C. §§ 2510-2522), or the Foreign Intelligence Surveillance Act, or Executive Order 12333 § 2.5.

B. (U//FOUO) Physical searches, including mail openings, in conformity with Rule 41 of the Federal Rules of Criminal Procedure, the Foreign Intelligence Surveillance Act, or Executive Order 12333 § 2.5. **Note:** For additional information regarding certain searches, see the classified appendix.

C. (U) Acquisition of foreign intelligence information in conformity with Title VII of the FISA.

(U//FOUO) **Note:** Not all investigative methods are authorized while collecting foreign intelligence as part of a full investigation. See DIOG Section 9 for more information.

11.2.4. (U) Particular Investigative Methods

(U//FOUO) All lawful investigative methods may be used in activities under the AGG-Dom as authorized by the AGG-Dom. Authorized methods include, but are not limited to, those identified in the rest of this section. In some instances they are subject to special restrictions or review or approval requirements. (AGG-Dom, Part V.A.)

11.3. (U) Investigative Method: Mail Covers

11.3.1.   (U) Summary

(U) A mail cover may be sought only in a predicated investigation when there exists reasonable grounds to demonstrate that the mail cover is necessary to: (i) protect the national security; (ii) locate a fugitive; (iii) obtain evidence of the commission or attempted commission of a federal crime; or (iv) assist in the identification of property, proceeds or assets forfeitable because of a violation of criminal law. 39 C.F.R. § 233.3(e)(2).

(U//FOUO)   b2
                                                                                                    b7E

(U)   b2
                                                                                                    b7E

As a general rule, a mail cover in the APO/FPO system overseas may only be ordered by a military authority competent to order searches and seizures for law enforcement purposes, usually a commanding officer. See DoD 4525.6-M, the DoD Postal Manual.

(U//FOUO) Application: b2
                                                                                                    b7E

11.3.2.   (U) Legal Authority

A. (U) Postal Service Regulation 39 C.F.R. § 233.3 is the sole authority and procedure for initiating a mail cover and for processing, using and disclosing information obtained from a mail cover;

B. (U) There is no Fourth Amendment protection for information on the outside of a piece of mail. See, e.g., U.S. v. Choate, 576 F.2d 165, 174 (9th Cir., 1978); and U.S. v. Huie, 593 F.2d 14 (5th Cir., 1979); and

C. (U) AGG-Dom, Part V.A.2.

11.3.3.   (U) Definition of Investigative Method

(U) A mail cover is the non-consensual recording of any data appearing on the outside cover of any sealed or unsealed mail matter to obtain information in order to:

A. (U) Protect the national security;

B. (U) Locate a fugitive;

C. (U) Obtain evidence of commission or attempted commission of a federal crime;

D. (U) Obtain evidence of a violation or attempted violation of a postal statute; or

E. (U) Assist in the identification of property, proceeds or assets forfeitable under law. 39 C.F.R. § 233.3(c) (1).

(U) In this context, a "recording" means the transcription, photograph, photocopy, or other facsimile of the image of the outside cover, envelope, or wrappers of mailed matter. A warrant or court order is almost always required to obtain the contents of any class of mail, sealed or unsealed.

11.3.4. (U) Standard for Use and Approval Requirements for Investigative Method

(U) The standard to obtain a mail cover is established by the Postal Service regulation. The Chief Postal Inspector may order a mail cover "[w]hen a written request is received from any law enforcement agency in which the requesting authority specifies the reasonable grounds to demonstrate the mail cover is necessary to:

- (U) Protect the national security;

- (U) Locate a fugitive;

- (U) Obtain information regarding the commission or attempted commission of a crime; or

- (U) Assist in the identification of property, proceeds or assets forfeitable because of a violation of criminal law." 29 C.F.R. § 233.3(e)(2).

(U/FOUO) **National Security Mail Cover:** A national security mail cover request must be approved by the Director or designee, currently only the EAD of the National Security Branch. All requests for national security mail covers must be reviewed by the Field Office SSA according to the below-criteria. A national security mail cover sought "to protect the national security" includes protecting the United States from actual or threatened attack or other grave, hostile act; sabotage; international terrorism; or clandestine intelligence activities, including commercial [economic] espionage by foreign powers or their agents.

(U//FOUO) After being approved by the SSA, the Field Office must transmit the mail cover letter request by EC, with the draft letter as an attachment, to the National Security Law Branch (NSLB) for legal review and concurrence. Upon review and concurrence, the NSLB must transmit the letter request for signature approval to the EAD, National Security Branch, or, in his or her absence, to the Director.

(U//FOUO) **Criminal Mail Cover:** A criminal mail cover request may be approved by the Field Office SSA. The SSA may approve a request for a mail cover if there are reasonable grounds to demonstrate that the mail cover is necessary to assist in efforts to: (i) locate a fugitive; (ii) obtain information regarding the commission or attempted commission of a federal crime; or (iii) to assist in the identification of property, proceeds or assets forfeitable because of a violation of criminal law.

(U//FOUO) **SSA review and or approval of a national security or criminal mail cover request:** Approval of any mail cover request or an extension is conditioned on the following criteria being met:

A. (U//FOUO)

b2
b7E

B. (U//FOUO)

b2
b7E

C. (U//FOUO)

b2
b7E

D. (U//FOUO)

b2
b7E

E. (U//FOUO)

b2
b7E

F. (U//FOUO) (Note:

b2
b7E

Under postal regulations, a mail cover must not include matter mailed between the mail cover subject and the subject's attorney, unless the attorney is also a subject under the investigation.)

b2
b7E

G. (U//FOUO)

b2
b7E

H. (U//FOUO)

b2
b7E

I. (U//FOUO)

b2
b7E

(U) **Emergency Requests:** When time is of the essence, the Chief Postal Inspector, or designee, may act upon an oral request to be confirmed by the requesting authority, in writing, within three calendar days. Information may be released prior to receipt of the written request only when the releasing official is satisfied that an emergency situation exists. 39 C.F.R. § 233.3(e)(3).

(U) An "emergency situation" exists when the immediate release of information is required to prevent the loss of evidence or when there is a potential for immediate physical harm to persons or property. 39 C.F.R. § 233.3(c)(10).

11.3.5. (U) Duration of Approval

A. (U) **National Security:** A national security mail cover is limited to 120 days from the date the mail cover is initiated. Extensions can only be authorized by the Chief Postal Inspector or his designee at the National Headquarters of the Office of the Chief Postal Inspector. 39 C.F.R. § 233.3(g)(6).

B. (U) **Criminal mail covers except fugitives:** A mail cover in a criminal case is limited to no more than 30 days, unless adequate justification is provided by the requesting authority. 39 C.F.R. § 233.3(g)(5). Renewals may be granted for additional 30-day periods under the same conditions and procedures applicable to the original request. The requesting authority must provide a statement of the investigative benefit of the mail cover and anticipated benefits to be derived from the extension.

C. (U) **Fugitives:** No mail cover instituted to locate a fugitive may remain in force for longer than 120 continuous days unless personally approved for further extension by the Chief Postal Inspector or his/her designees at National Headquarters. 39 C.F.R. § 233.3(g)(6).

D. (U) **Exception for Indictments:** Except for fugitive cases, no mail cover may remain in force when an information has been filed or the subject has been indicted for the matter for which the mail cover has been requested. If the subject is under investigation for further criminal violations, or a mail cover is required to assist in the identification of property, proceeds or assets forfeitable because of a violation of criminal law, a new mail cover order must be requested. 39 C.F.R. § 233.3(g)(7).

11.3.6. (U) Specific Procedures

(U//FOUO) The Postal Regulation requires that physical storage of all reports issued pursuant to a mail cover request to be at the discretion of the Chief Postal Inspector. 39 C.F.R. § 233.3(h)(1). Accordingly, FBI employees must conduct a timely review of mail cover documents received from the USPS. A copy of the signed mail cover request and the signed transmittal letter must be maintained in the investigative case file.

(U//FOUO)

b2
b7E

11.3.7. (U) Compliance and Monitoring

(U//FOUO) FBI employees must conduct a timely review of mail cover information received from the USPS for any potential production of data beyond the scope of the requested mail cover ("overproduction") and either destroy or return the overproduction to the assigned USPS representative noting the reason for the return.

11.4. **(U) Investigative Method: Physical searches of personal or real property where a warrant or court order is not legally required because there is no reasonable expectation of privacy (e.g.,** _____

b2
b7E

11.4.1. **(U) Summary**

(U//FOUO) **Application:** In predicated investigations, the FBI may conduct physical searches of personal or real property where a warrant or court order is not legally required because there is no reasonable expectation of privacy _____

b2
b7E

_____ not otherwise prohibited by AGG-Dom, Part III.B.2-3. _____

11.4.2. **(U) Legal Authority**

A. (U) AGG-Dom, Part V.A.3,

B. (U) Fourth Amendment to the United States Constitution

11.4.3. **(U) Definition of Investigative Method**

(U) The Fourth Amendment to the United States Constitution prevents the FBI from conducting unreasonable searches and seizures. It also generally requires a warrant be obtained if the search will intrude on a reasonable expectation of privacy. To qualify as a "reasonable expectation of privacy," the individual must have an actual subjective expectation of privacy and society must be prepared to recognize that expectation as objectively reasonable. See Katz v. United States, 389 U.S. at 361. If an individual has a reasonable expectation of privacy, a warrant or order issued by a court of competent jurisdiction or an exception to the requirement for such a warrant or order is required before a search may be conducted. Physical searches of personal or real property may be conducted without a search warrant or court order if there is no reasonable expectation of privacy in the property or area. As a general matter, there is no reasonable expectation of privacy in areas that are exposed to public view or that are otherwise available to the public. A reasonable expectation of privacy may be terminated by an individual abandoning property, setting trash at the edge of the curtilage or beyond for collection, or when a private party reveals the contents of a package.

(U) **Examples of Searches not Requiring a Warrant because there is no Reasonable Expectation of Privacy:** (i) Vehicle identification numbers or personal property that is exposed to public view and may be seen when looking through the window of a car that is parked in an area that is open to and accessible by members of the public; (ii) neither the examination of books and magazines in a book store nor the purchase of such items is a search or seizure under the Fourth Amendment. See Maryland v. Macon, 472 U.S. 463 (1985); and (iii) a deliberate overflight in navigable air space to photograph marijuana plants is not a search, despite the landowners subjective expectation of privacy. See California v. Ciraolo, 476 U.S. 207 (1986).

(U) Whether an area is curtilage is determined by reference to four factors: (i) proximity of the area in question to the home; (ii) whether the area is within an enclosure surrounding the home; (iii) nature of the use to which the area is put; and (iv) steps taken to protect the area from observation by passers-by.

(U) An area is curtilage if it "is so intimately tied to the home itself that it should be placed under the home's 'umbrella' of Fourth Amendment protection."

11.4.4. (U//FOUO) Standards for Use and Approval Requirements for Investigative Method

(U//FOUO) No supervisory approval is required for the use of this method. However, if there is a doubt as to whether a person has a reasonable expectation of privacy in the area to be searched, consult with the CDC or FBI Office of the General Counsel to determine whether a search warrant is required. Use of this method must be documented in the case file.

11.5. (U) Investigative Method: Consensual Monitoring of Communications, including consensual computer monitoring

11.5.1. (U) Summary

(U) Consensual monitoring of communications may be used in predicated investigations. Its use, including consensual computer monitoring, requires review by the CDC or the OGC. (AGG-Dom, Part V.A.4)

(U//FOUO) **Application:** This investigative method may be used in national security investigations, criminal investigations and positive foreign intelligence collection cases, and for assistance to other agencies when it is not otherwise prohibited by AGG-Dom, Part III.B.2-3. This method cannot be used during an assessment

(U//FOUO) **Note:** For those state, local and tribal governments that do not sanction or provide a law enforcement exception available to the FBI for one-party consensual recording of communications with persons within their jurisdiction, the SAC must approve the consensual monitoring of communications as an OIA. Prior to the SAC authorizing the OIA, one-party consent must be acquired. The SAC may delegate the OIA approval authority to an ASAC or SSA.

11.5.2. (U) Legal Authority

A. (U) The Fourth Amendment to the United States Constitution and case law interpreting the same;

B. (U) 18 U.S.C. § 2511(2)(b) & (c);

C. (U) The Foreign Intelligence Surveillance Act of 1978 (FISA), 50 U.S.C. §§ 1801 et seq., defines "electronic surveillance" to include only those communications "in which a person has a reasonable expectation of privacy and a warrant would be required for law enforcement purposes." 50 U.S.C. § 1801(f). If a party to the communication has consented to monitoring, a Title III or FISA court order is not required to monitor those consensual communications; and

D. (U) Computer Trespasser Exception - 18 U.S.C. § 2511(2)(i).

11.5.3. (U) Definition of Investigative Method

(U) Consensual monitoring is: "monitoring of communications for which a court order or warrant is not legally required because of the consent of a party to the communication." (AGG-Dom, Part VII.A.) Consensual monitoring includes the interception of the content of communications that typically fall into one of three general categories:

A. (U) Conventional telephone communications or other means of transmitting the human voice through cable, wire, radio frequency (RF), or other similar connections;

B. (U) Oral communications, typically intercepted through the use of devices that monitor and record oral conversations (e.g., where a body transmitter or recorder or a fixed location transmitter or recorder is used during a face-to-face communication in which a person would have a reasonable expectation of privacy but for the consent of the other party); and

C. (U) Communications transmitted between parties using computer protocols, such as e-mail, instant message, chat sessions, text messaging, peer-to-peer communications, or other "electronic communications," as that term is defined in 18 U.S.C. § 2510(12).

(U) The consensual monitoring of communications, including consensual computer monitoring, is subject to legal review by the CDC or the OGC. (AGG-Dom, Part V.A.4)

(U) The computer trespasser exception to the wiretap statute, 18 U.S.C. § 2511(2)(i), relies on the consent of the computer owner-operator and limits the monitoring to only the communications of the trespasser. The statute includes additional limitations on the use of this provision.

11.5.4. (U) Standards for Use and Approval Requirements for Investigative Method

A. (U) General Approval Requirements

(U//FOUO) Except as provided below in Section 11.5.4.B, an SSA may approve the consensual monitoring of communications, including consensual computer monitoring of communications, if the information likely to be obtained is relevant to an ongoing investigation. SSA approval is conditioned on the following criteria being met and documented using the FD-759:

1. (U//FOUO) **Reasons for Monitoring:** There is sufficient factual information supporting the need for the monitoring and that the monitoring is related to the investigative purpose, including, if applicable, a citation to the principal criminal statute involved;

2. (U//FOUO) **Legal Review:** Prior to the initiation of the consensual monitoring, the CDC or the OGC concurred that consensual monitoring under the facts of the investigation is legal. Whenever the monitoring circumstances change substantially, a new FD-759 must be executed and the CDC or OGC must be recontacted to obtain a new concurrence. (AGG-Dom, Part V.A.4.) The following are examples of substantial changes in monitoring circumstances which require a new FD-759: a different consenting party, new interceptees, or a change in the location of a fixed monitoring device.

3. (U) **Consent:** A party to the communication has consented to the monitoring and that consent has been documented according to the below procedures. Consent may be express or implied. In consensual computer monitoring, for example, implied consent to monitor may exist if users are given notice through a sign-on banner that all users must actively acknowledge (by clicking through) or through other means of obvious notice of possible monitoring. Consent to monitor pursuant to the computer trespasser exception is not provided by a party to the communication per se, but is instead provided by the owner, operator, or systems administrator of the computer to be monitored.

4. (U//FOUO) **Subject:** The monitoring will not intentionally include a third-party who is not of interest to the investigation, except for unavoidable or inadvertent overhears.

5. (U//FOUO) **Location of device:** Appropriate safeguards exist to ensure that the consenting party remains a party to the communication throughout the course of monitoring. If a fixed-location monitoring device is being used, the consenting party

has been admonished and agrees to be present during the duration of the monitoring and, if practicable, technical means are being used to activate monitoring only when the consenting party is present.

6. (U//FOUO) **Location of monitoring:** If monitoring will occur outside a Field Office's territory, notice has been provided to the SAC or ASAC of each Field Office where the monitoring is to occur, and that notice has been documented in the case file.

7. (U//FOUO) **Duration:** The request states the length of time needed for monitoring. Unless otherwise warranted, approval may be granted for the duration of the investigation subject to a substantial change of circumstances, as described in Section 11.5.4.A.2, above. When a "sensitive monitoring circumstance" is involved, DOJ may limit its approval to a shorter duration.

B. (U//FOUO) **Exceptions Requiring Additional Approval**

1. (U//FOUO) <u>Party Located Outside the United States:</u>

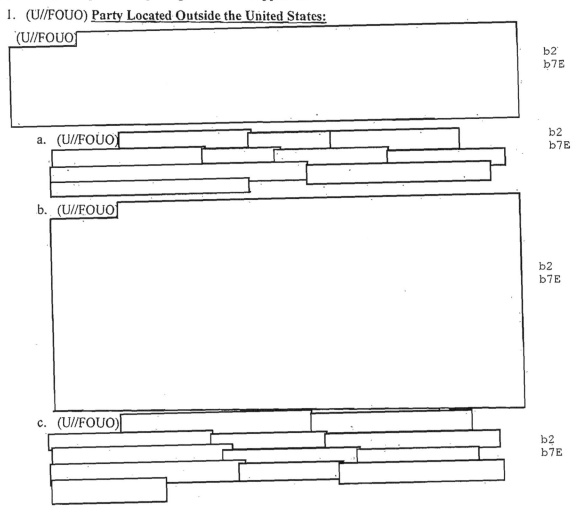

(U//FOUO)   b2
                                                                            b7E

a. (U//FOUO)   b2
                                                                           b7E

b. (U//FOUO)   b2
                                                                           b7E

c. (U//FOUO)   b2
                                                                           b7E

2. (U) **Consent of More than One Party Required:**

(U//FOUO) For those states or tribes that do not sanction or provide a law enforcement exception available to the FBI for one-party consent recording of communications with persons within their jurisdiction, the SAC must approve the consensual monitoring of communications as an OIA. Prior to the SAC authorizing the OIA, one-party consent must be acquired. The SAC may delegate the OIA approval authority to an ASAC or SSA.

3. (U) **Sensitive Monitoring Circumstance:**

(U) Requests to consensually monitor communications when a sensitive monitoring circumstance is involved must be approved by the DOJ Criminal Division, or if the investigation concerns a threat to the national security or foreign intelligence collection, by the DOJ NSD. (AGG-Dom, Part V.A.4) A "sensitive monitoring circumstance" is defined in the AGG-Dom, Part VII.O, to include the following:

a. (U) Investigation of a member of Congress, a federal judge, a member of the Executive Branch at Executive Level IV or above, or a person who has served in such capacity within the previous two years (**Note:** Executive Levels I through IV are defined in 5 U.S.C. §§ 5312-5315);

b. (U) Investigation of the Governor, Lieutenant Governor, or Attorney General of any state or territory, or a judge or justice of the highest court of any state or territory, concerning an offense involving bribery, conflict of interest, or extortion related to the performance of official duties;

c. (U) The Attorney General, the Deputy Attorney General, or an Assistant Attorney General has requested that the FBI obtain prior approval for the use of consensual monitoring in a specific investigation;

d. (U) A party to the communication is in the custody of the Bureau of Prisons or the United States Marshal Service or is being or has been afforded protection in the Witness Security Program.

(U//FOUO)

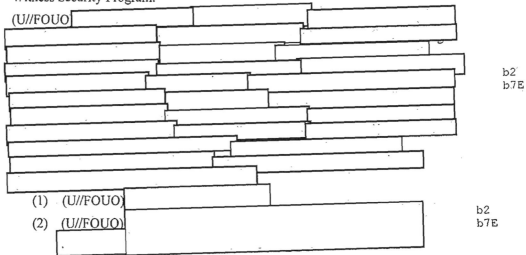

b2
b7E

(1) (U//FOUO)

(2) (U//FOUO)

b2
b7E

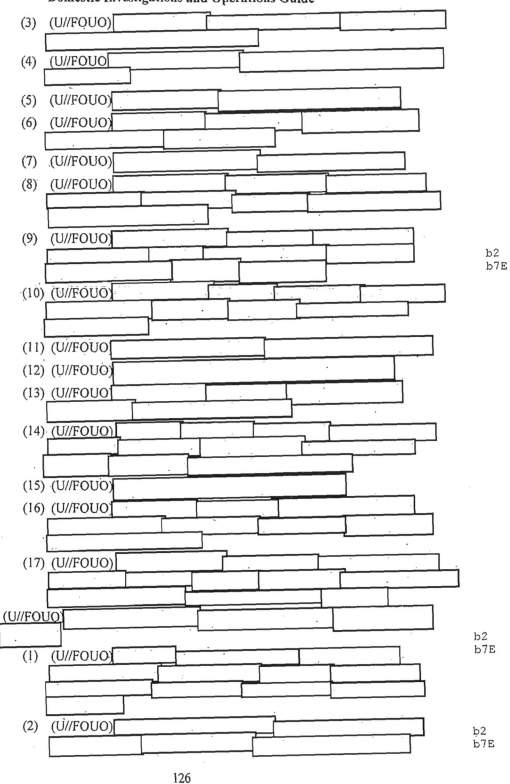

(3) (U//FOUO)

(4) (U//FOUO

(5) (U//FOUO)

(6) (U//FOUO)

(7) (U//FOUO)

(8) (U//FOUO)

(9) (U//FOUO)

b2
b7E

(10) (U//FOUO)

(11) (U//FOUO

(12) (U//FOUO)

(13) (U//FOUO

(14) (U//FOUO)

(15) (U//FOUO)

(16) (U//FOUO)

(17) (U//FOUO)

(U//FOUO)

b2
b7E

(1) (U//FOUO)

(2) (U//FOUO)

b2
b7E

(U//FOUO) **Note:** See classified <u>Appendix G</u> for additional information regarding consensual monitoring.

e. (U//FOUO) **Procedure for Obtaining DOJ Approval For a Sensitive Monitoring Circumstance:**

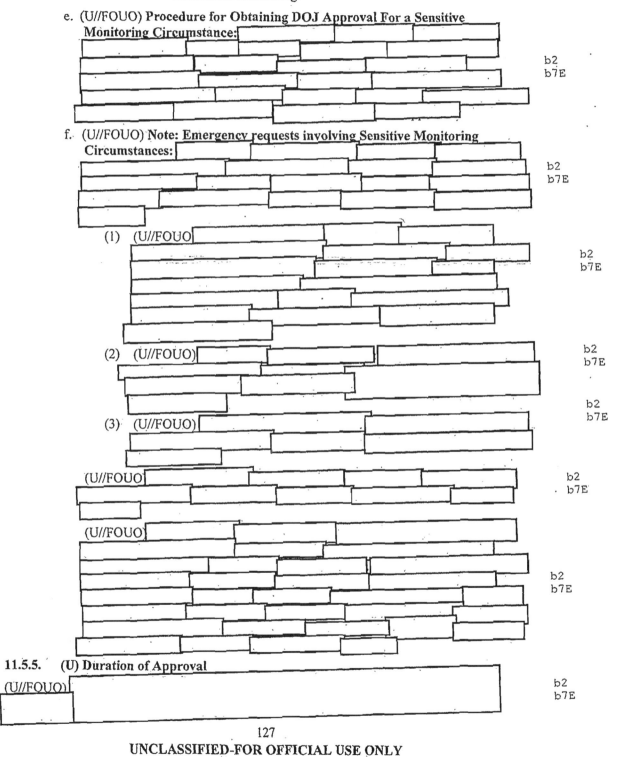

b2
b7E

f. (U//FOUO) **Note: Emergency requests involving Sensitive Monitoring Circumstances:**

b2
b7E

    (1) (U//FOUO

b2
b7E

    (2) (U//FOUO)

b2
b7E

b2
b7E

    (3) (U//FOUO)

(U//FOUO

b2
b7E

(U//FOUO)

b2
b7E

11.5.5.   **(U) Duration of Approval**

(U//FOUO)

b2
b7E

b2
b7E

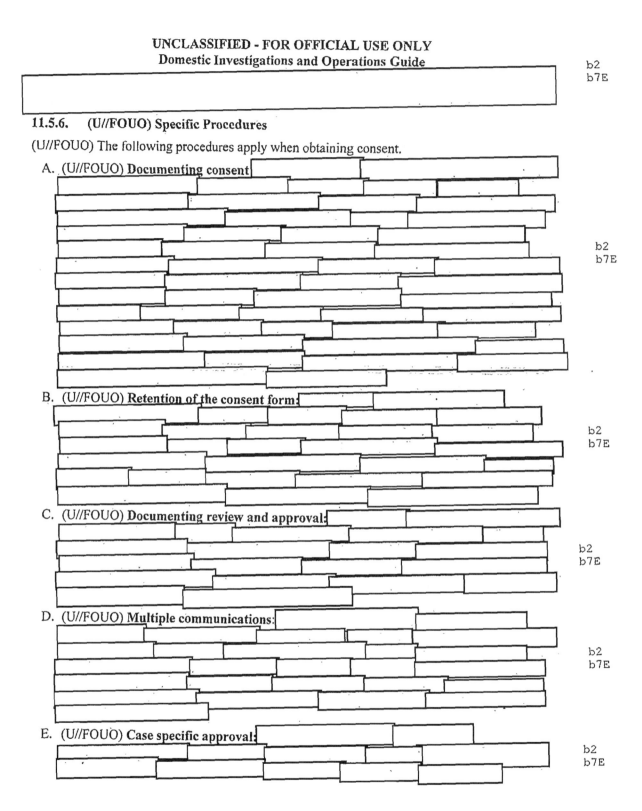

11.5.6. **(U//FOUO) Specific Procedures**

(U//FOUO) The following procedures apply when obtaining consent.

A. (U//FOUO) **Documenting consent**

b2
b7E

B. (U//FOUO) **Retention of the consent form:**

b2
b7E

C. (U//FOUO) **Documenting review and approval:**

b2
b7E

D. (U//FOUO) **Multiple communications:**

b2
b7E

E. (U//FOUO) **Case specific approval:**

b2
b7E

11.5.7. (U//FOUO) Compliance and Monitoring

(U//FOUO) ELSUR program personnel must conduct regularly scheduled reviews of the FD-759s approved within the Field Office to determine whether approval was obtained prior to initiation of consensual monitoring and to ensure that the monitoring occurred in compliance with the approvals. The ELSUR Program is also responsible for indexing all individuals or identifiers of persons intercepted during consensual monitoring and cross-referencing their names or identifiers to the approved FD-759 in the investigative case file.

11.6. (U) Investigative Method: Use of closed-circuit television, direction finders, and other monitoring devices (Not needing a Court Order)

(U) Note: Use of this method is subject to legal review by the CDC or OGC.

11.6.1. (U) Summary

(U//FOUO)

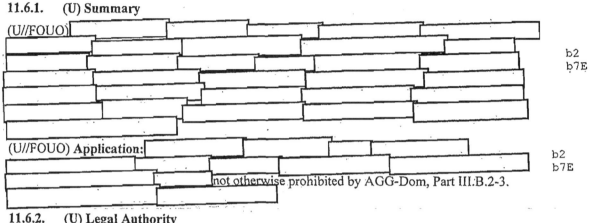

b2
b7E

(U//FOUO) Application:

not otherwise prohibited by AGG-Dom, Part III.B.2-3.

b2
b7E

11.6.2. (U) Legal Authority

A. (U) AGG-Dom, Part V

B. (U) Tracking devices use (18 U.S.C. § 2510[12] [C])

C. (U) Rule 41 Federal Rules of Criminal Procedure

D. (U) Fourth Amendment to the United States Constitution

11.6.3. (U//FOUO) Definition of Investigative Method

A. (U//FOUO) Closed Circuit Television (CCTV): a fixed-location video camera that is typically concealed from view or that is placed on or operated by a consenting party.

B. (U//FOUO) Electronic Tracking Devices:

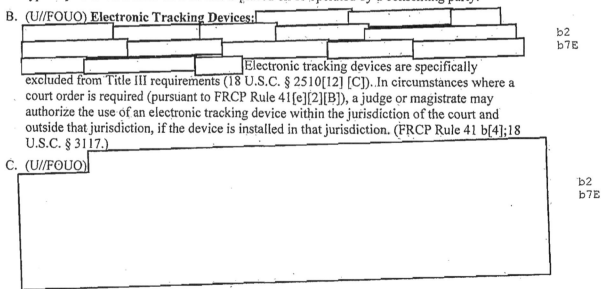

b2
b7E

Electronic tracking devices are specifically excluded from Title III requirements (18 U.S.C. § 2510[12] [C]). In circumstances where a court order is required (pursuant to FRCP Rule 41[e][2][B]), a judge or magistrate may authorize the use of an electronic tracking device within the jurisdiction of the court and outside that jurisdiction, if the device is installed in that jurisdiction. (FRCP Rule 41 b[4];18 U.S.C. § 3117.)

C. (U//FOUO)

b2
b7E

(U//FOUO)

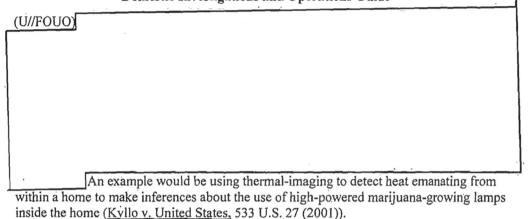

An example would be using thermal-imaging to detect heat emanating from within a home to make inferences about the use of high-powered marijuana-growing lamps inside the home (Kyllo v. United States, 533 U.S. 27 (2001)).

(U) Whether an area is curtilage is determined by reference to four factors: (i) proximity of the area in question to the home; (ii) whether the area is within an enclosure surrounding the home; (iii) nature of the use to which the area is put; and (iv) steps taken to protect the area from observation by passers-by.

11.6.4. (U//FOUO) Standards for Use and Approval Requirements for Investigative Method

(U//FOUO) When a video camera is physically operated as a hand-held video and is being used in an area in which no one has a reasonable expectation of privacy, its use is equivalent to using a still camera and does not require supervisory approval.

(U//FOUO) For those situations that require SSA approval for the use of CCTV, tracking devices, and other monitoring devices, SSA approval, which should be documented using the FD-759, may be granted if the following criteria have been met:

A. (U//FOUO) Legal review and concurrence from the CDC or OGC that a court order is not required for installation or use of the device because there has been lawful consent, no reasonable expectation of privacy exists, or no physical trespass necessary to install the device. **Note:** Whenever circumstances change in either installation or monitoring, a new legal review should be obtained to determine whether a separate authorization is necessary.

B. (U//FOUO) Use of the method is reasonably likely to achieve investigative objectives:

C. (U//FOUO)

D. (U//FOUO)

  1. (U//FOUO)

  2. (U//FOUO

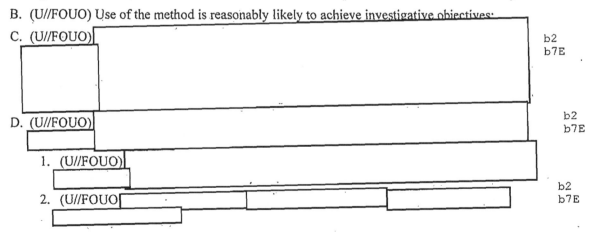

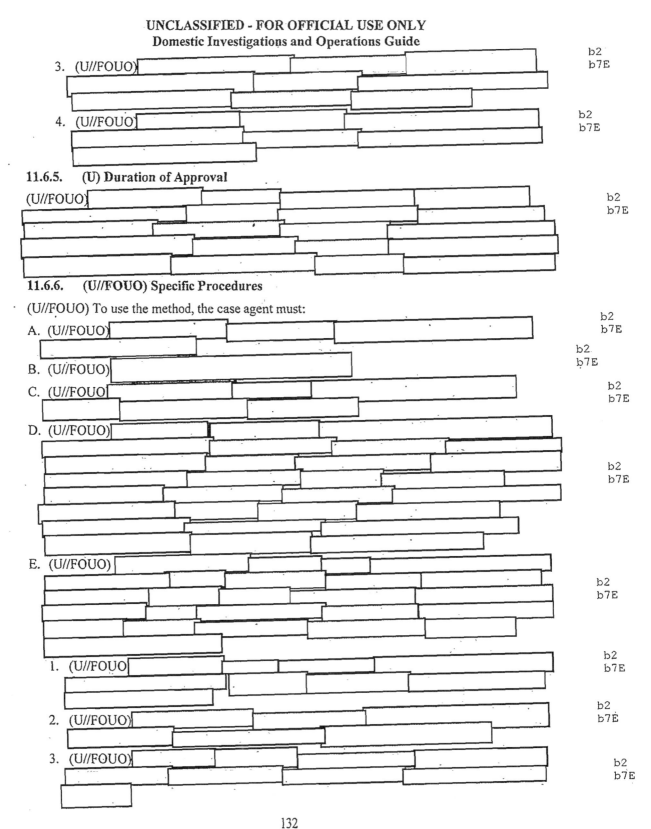

3. (U//FOUO)   b2
                                                                       b7E

4. (U//FOUO)   b2
                                                                       b7E

11.6.5.   (U) Duration of Approval

(U//FOUO)   b2
                                                                       b7E

11.6.6.   (U//FOUO) Specific Procedures

(U//FOUO) To use the method, the case agent must: b2
                                                                       b7E
A. (U//FOUO)

                                                                       b2
                                                                       b7E
B. (U//FOUO)

C. (U//FOUO)   b2
                                                                       b7E

D. (U//FOUO)

                                                                       b2
                                                                       b7E

E. (U//FOUO)

                                                                       b2
                                                                       b7E

1. (U//FOUO)   b2
                                                                       b7E

2. (U//FOUO)   b2
                                                                       b7E

3. (U//FOUO)   b2
                                                                       b7E

(U//FOUO) [redacted]   b2
                                                        b7E

11.6.7.   (U//FOUO) Compliance and Monitoring

(U//FOUO) Authorization documents regarding the use of the CCTV, electronic tracking devices   b2
[redacted] must be documented in the substantive investigative ELSUR file   b7E
and will be available for compliance and monitoring review.

11.7. (U) Investigative Method: Polygraph

11.7.1. (U) Summary

(U//FOUO) Application:

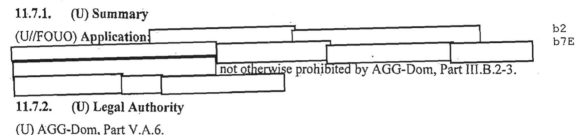

not otherwise prohibited by AGG-Dom, Part III.B.2-3.

b2
b7E

11.7.2. (U) Legal Authority

(U) AGG-Dom, Part V.A.6.

11.7.3. (U//FOUO) Definition of Investigative Method

(U//FOUO) The polygraph is used to: (i) aid in determining whether a person has pertinent knowledge of a particular matter under investigation or inquiry; (ii) aid in determining the truthfulness of statements made or information furnished by a subject, victim, witness, CHS, or an individual making allegations; (iii) obtain information leading to the location of evidence, individuals or sites of offense; and (iv) assist in verifying the accuracy and thoroughness of information furnished by applicants and employees.

(U//FOUO)

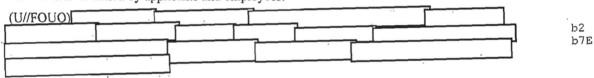

b2
b7E

(U//FOUO) **Note:** This policy does not limit other authorized activities of the FBI, such as the FBI's responsibilities to conduct background checks and inquiries concerning applicants and employees under federal personnel security programs.

11.7.4. (U//FOUO) Standards for Use and Approval Requirements for Investigative Method

(U//FOUO) An SSA may approve the use of a polygraph if:

A. (U//FOUO)

B. (U//FOUO)

C. (U//FOUO)

b2
b7E

11.7.5. (U) Duration of Approval

(U//FOUO)

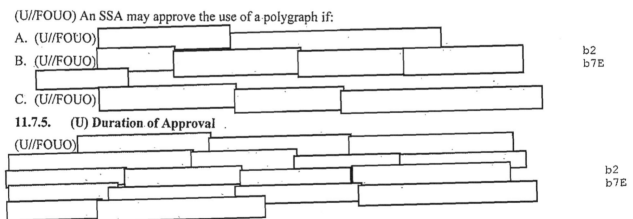

b2
b7E

11.7.6. (U//FOUO) Specific Procedures

(U//FOUO) An EC must be prepared requesting SSA approval for the polygraph. If an AUSA is assigned to the case, an FBI employee must confer with the USAO to discuss any prosecutorial issues prior to the administration of a polygraph.

11.7.7. (U//FOUO) Compliance and Monitoring

(U//FOUO) Except for polygraphs administered as part of a background check or as part of a federal personnel security program, all polygraphs must be conducted under and documented to a substantive case file.

11.8. (U) Investigative Method: Undercover Operations

11.8.1. (U) Summary

(U//FOUO)

b2
b7E

(U//FOUO) Undercover operations must be conducted in conformity with *The Attorney General's Guidelines on Federal Bureau of Investigation Undercover Operations* (AGG-UCO) in investigations relating to activities in violation of federal criminal law that do not concern threats to the national security or foreign intelligence. In investigations that concern threats to the national security or foreign intelligence, undercover operations involving religious or political organizations must be reviewed and approved by FBI Headquarters, with participation by the NSD in the review process. (AGG-Dom, Part V.A.7) Other undercover operations involving threats to the national security or foreign intelligence are reviewed and approved pursuant to FBI policy as described herein.

(U//FOUO) **Application:**

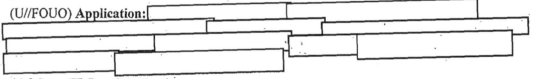

b2
b7E

11.8.2. (U) Legal Authority

A. (U) AGG-Dom, Part V.A.7

B. (U) AGG-UCO

11.8.3. (U//FOUO) Definition of Investigative Method

A. (U//FOUO) An "undercover activity" is any investigative activity involving the use of an assumed identity by an undercover employee for an official purpose, investigative activity, or function. An "undercover employee" is an employee of the FBI, another federal, state, or local law enforcement agency, another entity of the United States Intelligence Community, or another foreign intelligence agency working under the direction and control of the FBI whose relationship with the FBI is concealed from third parties by the maintenance of a cover or alias identity for an official purpose, investigative activity, or function.

B. (U//FOUO) An "undercover operation" is an operation that involves a series of related "undercover activities" over a period of time by an "undercover employee." A series of related undercover activities consists of more than five separate substantive contacts by an undercover employee with the individuals under investigation. In investigations relating to activities in violation of federal criminal law that do not concern threats to the national security or foreign intelligence, undercover activity involving sensitive circumstances, which are listed in the AGG-UCO and the FGUSO, constitutes an undercover operation regardless of the number of contacts involved. A substantive contact is a communication, whether by

136

oral, written, wire, or electronic means, that includes information of investigative interest. Mere incidental contact (e.g., a conversation that establishes an agreed time and location for another meeting) is not a substantive contact within the meaning of this policy.

(U//FOUO) Distinction Between Sensitive Circumstance and Sensitive Investigative Matter:

(U//FOUO) The term "sensitive investigative matter" as used in the AGG-Dom should not be confused with the term "sensitive circumstance" as that term is used in undercover operations or ELSUR matters. The term sensitive circumstance relates to a circumstance that arises in an undercover operation that requires the UCO to obtain FBIHQ approval. A comprehensive list of sensitive circumstances for criminal activities is contained in the AGG-UCO and for national security matters in Section 28 of the NFIPM. The Criminal Undercover Operations Review Committee (CUORC) and the national security Undercover Review Committee (UCRC) must review and approve undercover operations that involve sensitive circumstances. The detailed policy for undercover operations is described in this section of the DIOG, the Field Guide for Undercover and Sensitive Operations (FGUSO), and the FBIHQ substantive Division program implementation guides.

11.8.4. (U//FOUO) Standards for Use and Approval Requirements for Investigative Method

A. (U//FOUO) An official considering approval or authorization of a proposed undercover application must weigh the risks and benefits of the operation, giving careful consideration to the following:

1. (U//FOUO) The risks of personal injury to individuals, property damage, financial loss to persons or business, damage to reputation, or other harm to persons;

2. (U//FOUO) The risk of civil liability or other loss to the government;

3. (U//FOUO) The risk of invasion of privacy or interference with privileged or confidential relationships and any potential constitutional concerns or other legal concerns;

4. (U//FOUO) The risk that individuals engaged in undercover operations may become involved in illegal conduct;

5. (U//FOUO) The suitability of government participation in the type of activity that is expected to occur during the operation. (AGG-UCO, Part IV.A.)

B. (U//FOUO) The following approval and authorization requirements apply to undercover operations relating to activities in violation of federal criminal law that do not concern threats to the national security or foreign intelligence:

1. (U//FOUO) An "undercover activity" in which an undercover employee plans to meet with a subject requires the approval of the SSA.

2. (U//FOUO) An "undercover operation" must be approved by the SAC (or an ASAC with delegated approval authority). The CDC must review all undercover operations before approval and provide advice to the SAC regarding predication of subjects, entrapment issues, and whether the proposal meets the requirements of the AGG-UCO or other DOJ and FBI policy guidance.

3. (U//FOUO) In addition to SAC approval, authorization from the responsible FBIHQ Assistant Director or Executive Assistant Director must be obtained if the undercover operation involves a sensitive circumstance or certain fiscal circumstances, as those terms are defined in the AGG-UCO or other FBI guidance.

4. (U//FOUO) Undercover operations that involve a sensitive circumstance (Group I undercover operations) require review by the CUORC as part of the authorization process. This requirement applies to both new and renewal proposals.

5. (U//FOUO) Undercover operations that do not involve a sensitive circumstance (Group II undercover operations) require notice to the appropriate FBIHQ substantive Unit and to the Undercover and Sensitive Operations Unit following SAC approval. A renewal that would extend the operation beyond one year requires authorization from the responsible Assistant Director.

6. (U//FOUO) All Innocent Images National Initiative (IINI) undercover operations deemed Group I and Group II operations require initiation and renewal approvals from FBIHQ, Cyber Division. Group I IINI undercover operations will also be reviewed by the CUORC.

7. (U//FOUO) Requirements for interim approval and emergency approval for undercover operations are contained in the FGUSO.

C. (U//FOUO) The following approval requirements apply to undercover operations that concern threats to the national security or foreign intelligence:

1. (U//FOUO) An "undercover operation" must be approved by the SAC (or an ASAC with delegated approval authority). The CDC must review all undercover operations before approval and provide advice to the SAC regarding predication of subjects, entrapment issues, and whether the proposal meets the requirements of Section 28 of the NFIPM, or its successor, or other DOJ and FBI policy guidance.

2. (U//FOUO) In addition to SAC approval, authorization from the responsible FBIHQ Assistant Director or Executive Assistant Director must be obtained if the undercover operation involves a sensitive circumstance, as defined in Section 28 of the NFIPM, or its successor.

3. (U//FOUO) Undercover operations that involve a sensitive circumstance must be reviewed and authorized by the responsible Assistant Director (Group I operations). Review by the UCRC must precede such authorization. If the matter involves religious or political organizations, the review must include participation by a representative of the DOJ NSD. (AGG-Dom, Section V; Section 28 of the NFIPM, or its successor)

4. (U//FOUO) Undercover operations that do not involve a sensitive circumstance (Group II undercover operations) must be forwarded to the appropriate substantive Unit at FBIHQ for review on a UACB basis prior to initiation of the operation. A renewal that would extend the operation beyond 12 months requires authorization from the responsible Deputy Assistant Director or Assistant Director.

5. (U//FOUO) Requirements for interim approval and emergency approval for undercover operations are contained in Section 28 of the NFIPM, or its successor.

11.8.5. **(U) Duration of Approval**

(U//FOUO)

b2
b7E

11.8.6. **(U) Additional Guidance**

A. (U//FOUO)

b2
b7E

B. (U//FOUO)

b2
b7E

C. (U//FOUO)

b2
b7E

11.8.7. **(U//FOUO) Compliance and Monitoring, and Reporting Requirements**

(U//FOUO) All UCOs must provide an _____ summary using the _____ to appropriate _____

b2
b7E

11.9. **(U) Investigative Method: Compulsory process as authorized by law, including grand jury subpoenas and other subpoenas, National Security Letters**

15 U.S.C. §§ 1681u, 1681v; 18 U.S.C. § 2709; 12 U.S.C. § 3414(a)(5)(A); 50 U.S.C. § 436, and FISA orders (50 U.S.C. §§ 1861-63).

(U) Summary

(U//FOUO)

b2
b7E

(U//FOUO) Application:

b2
b7E

When collecting positive foreign intelligence, if the subject is a non-United States person, a request for business records pursuant to 50 U.S.C. §§ 1861-63 is lawful.

11.9.1. **(U) Federal Grand Jury Subpoena**

A. **(U) Legal Authorities**

(U) A Federal Grand Jury is an independent panel charged with determining whether there is probable cause to believe one or more persons committed a particular federal offense within the venue of the district court. If the FGJ believes probable cause exists, it will vote a "true bill" and the person will be indicted. An FGJ indictment is the most typical way persons are charged with felonies in federal court. A FGJ can collect evidence through the use of an FGJ subpoena, which is governed by Rule 6 of the FRCP. FRCP 6(e) controls the release of information obtained by the prosecutor as part of the FGJ proceeding. FRCP 6(e) allows federal prosecutors to share valuable foreign intelligence, counterintelligence, and terrorism-related threat information, and it is the DOJ's policy that such information should be shared to the fullest extent permissible by law and in a manner consistent with the rule. The Attorney General has issued revised Guidelines for the Disclosure and Use of Grand Jury Information under Rule 6(e)(3)(D) (hereinafter "FGJ-Guidelines"). A memorandum issued by the Deputy Attorney General on May 15, 2008, provides amplifying guidance.

B. (U//FOUO) **Definition of Method**

(U//FOUO) FGJ subpoenas are demands for documents, records, testimony of witnesses, or any other evidence deemed relevant by a sitting grand jury. The FBI can request the issuance of an FGJ subpoena in coordination with the responsible United States Attorney's Office in all criminal investigative matters

b2
b7E

FGJ subpoenas are limited to use prior to the indictment of the individual to whom the subpoena relates.

C. (U) **Approval Requirements**

(U) There are no FBI supervisory approval requirements, but all FGJ subpoenas must be issued by the United States Attorney's Office that is handling the assessment or investigation to which the subpoenaed materials or witnesses are relevant.

D. (U) **Duration of Approval**

(U) FGJ subpoenas include a "return date," which is the date on which the subpoenaed materials or testimony is due to the grand jury.

E. (U) **Specific Procedures**

(U) FGJ subpoenas are governed by Rule 6(e) of the Federal Rules for Criminal Procedure and can only be obtained in coordination with the responsible United States Attorney's Office or the appropriate DOJ Division.

(U) **Note:** 28 C.F.R. § 50.10 requires the approval of the Attorney General before a trial or FGJ subpoena may be issued to a third party to obtain the telephone toll records of a member of the news media. Specific justification is required. Coordination with the Assistant United States Attorney handling the grand jury presentation or trial is necessary. Before proposing such a subpoena, an agent should review 28 C.F.R. § 50.10.

F. (U) **Notice and Reporting Requirements**

(U) There are no FBI notice or reporting requirements for FGJ subpoenas.

G. (U) **Grand Jury Proceedings—Generally**

1. (U) **Procedural Issues and Handling of FGJ Materials**

(U) The FGJ makes its determination whether to return a "true bill of indictment" based on evidence presented by the prosecuting attorney in an ex parte proceeding. The grand jury operates under the direction and guidance of the United States District Court. Generally, only witnesses for the prosecution testify before the grand jury.

(U) Only the United States Attorney or an assistant, other DOJ attorneys prosecuting the matter, the witness under examination, an interpreter (as needed), and the stenographer or operator of a recording device may be present while the grand jury is in session. No judge is present during the presentation of evidence although the court will sometime rule on evidentiary issues and will provide initial instructions to the FGJ. No person other than the grand jurors may be present while the grand jury is deliberating or voting.

2. (U) Restrictions on Disclosure

(U) As a general rule, no one other than a grand jury witness may disclose matters occurring before the grand jury. Government agents, even if called as witnesses, may not disclose matters occurring before the grand jury.

3. (U) Exceptions Permitting Disclosure

   a. (U) Disclosures by the government without the court's permission. The government, through its attorney, may disclose grand jury matters under the following conditions:

      i. (U) Under Rule 6(e)(3)(A), the government may disclose a grand jury matter to the following persons and in the following situations provided the government does not disclose the grand jury's deliberations or any grand juror's vote and the government provides the court that impaneled the grand jury with the names of all persons to whom disclosure was made and certifies that the government has advised the receiving party of the obligation of secrecy under this rule.

         (U) Persons eligible to receive material under this subsection are: 1) an attorney for the government for use in performing that attorney's duty; 2) any government personnel, including state, local, Indian tribe, or foreign government personnel that an attorney for the government considers necessary to assist in performing that attorney's duty to enforce federal law; and 3) a person authorized under 18 U.S.C. § 3322.

         (U) Note: FBI OGC attorneys and CDCs are not "attorneys for the government." Under this Rule, FRCP 1 defines "attorney for the government" as "the Attorney General, an authorized assistant of the Attorney General, a United States Attorney, [and] an authorized assistant of the United States Attorney."

      ii. (U) An attorney for the government may disclose any grand jury matter to another Federal Grand Jury.

iii. (U) An attorney for the government may disclose any grand jury matter involving foreign intelligence, counterintelligence, or foreign intelligence information to any federal law enforcement, intelligence, protective, immigration, national defense, or national security official to assist the official receiving the information in the performance of that official's duties. The government attorney must file, under seal, with the court that impaneled the grand jury, a notice that such information was disclosed and the agencies or departments that received the information. As used in Rule 6(e), foreign intelligence information is information that relates to the ability of the United States to protect against actual or potential attack or grave hostile acts by a foreign power or its agents; sabotage or international terrorism by a foreign power or its agents or clandestine intelligence activities by an intelligence service or network of a foreign power or its agents, or information with respect to a foreign power or foreign territory that relates to the national defense or security of the United States or the United States conduct of foreign affairs.

iv. (U) An attorney for the government may disclose any grand jury matter involving, either in the United States or elsewhere, a threat of attack or other grave hostile acts of a foreign power or its agent, a threat of domestic or international sabotage, or clandestine intelligence gathering activities by an intelligence service or network of a foreign power or by its agent to any appropriate federal, state, local, Indian tribal, or foreign government official for the purpose of preventing or responding to such threat or activities. The government attorney must file, under seal, with the court that impaneled the grand jury, a notice that such information was disclosed and the agencies or departments that received the information.

b. (U) **Disclosures by the government requiring the Court's permission.** The government, through its attorney, may disclose grand jury matters under the following conditions only with permission of the court. Petitions to make these disclosures are generally, but not always, filed with the court that impaneled the grand jury. Unless the hearing on the government's petition is to be ex parte, the petition must be served on all parties to the proceedings and the parties must be afforded a reasonable period of time to respond.

i. (U) An attorney for the government may petition for disclosure to a foreign court or prosecutor for use in an official criminal investigation.

ii. (U) An attorney for the government may petition for disclosure to a state, local, Indian tribal, or foreign government official, if the government attorney can show that the matter may disclose a violation of state, Indian tribal, or foreign criminal law, and the purpose of the disclosure is to enforce that law.

iii. (U) An attorney for the government may petition for disclosure to an appropriate military official if the government attorney can show the matter may disclose a violation of military criminal law under the Uniform Code of Military Justice, and the purpose of the disclosure is to enforce that law.

c. (U//FOUO) **FBI's Conduit Rule**

(U//FOUO) Only the federal prosecutor is authorized to make an initial disclosure of Rule 6(e)(3)(D) foreign intelligence information. As a practical matter, such disclosures are ordinarily accomplished through the FBI, which may have existing information-sharing mechanisms with authorized receiving officials. If the prosecutor intends to share information directly with another official, consultation with the FBI is required to ensure that disclosures will be consistent with the existing policy of intelligence community agencies and to ensure appropriate handling of sensitive or classified information.

b2
b7E

(U//FOUO) If, in cases of emergency, the prosecutor must disclose information before consulting with the FBI, the prosecutor must notify the FBI as soon as practicable.

d. (U) **Other Limitations**

(U) Rule 6(e)(3)(D) does not eliminate certain other information protection requirements, such as restrictions on disclosures of tax returns, on certain financial information under the Right to Financial Privacy Act, and on classified information, to name only a few examples. Specific statutes may impose additional burdens of disclosures.

e. (U) **Disclosure**

i. (U) An FBI employee may become a "Receiving Official," the person to whom grand jury information has been disclosed, if the FBI receives grand jury information developed during investigations conducted by other agencies. A Receiving Official is any federal, state, local, Indian tribal, or foreign government official receiving grand jury information, disclosed by an attorney for the government, under any provision of Rule 6(e)(3)(D). A Receiving Official may only use the disclosed material as necessary in the conduct of his/her official duties. The Receiving Official ordinarily must consult with the federal prosecutor before disseminating the information publicly, including in open court proceedings.

ii. (U//FOUO) Receiving Officials may only use grand jury information in a manner consistent with the FGJ-Guidelines and any additional conditions placed on the use or handling of grand jury information by the attorney for the government.

iii. (U//FOUO) If dissemination is necessary to the performance of his or her official duties, a Receiving Official may disseminate Rule 6(e)(3)(D) information outside of that official's agency to other government officials.

iv. (U) A Receiving Official, other than a foreign government official, must consult with the attorney for the government before disseminating Rule 6(e)(3)(D) information publicly (including through its use in a court proceeding that is open to or accessible to the public), unless prior dissemination is necessary to prevent harm to life or property. In such instances, the Receiving Official shall notify the attorney for the government of the dissemination as soon as practicable.

v. (U) A foreign government Receiving Official must obtain the prior consent from the disclosing official where possible, or if the disclosing is unavailable, from the agency that disseminated the information to that foreign official before dissemination of the information to a third government or publicly. Public dissemination includes using the information in a court proceeding that is open to or accessible by the public.

vi. (U) A Receiving Official shall handle Rule 6(e)(3)(D) information in a manner consistent with its sensitivity and shall take appropriate measures to restrict access to this information to individuals who require access for the performance of official duties.

vii. (U) A Receiving Official shall immediately report to the disclosing attorney for the government: any unauthorized dissemination of Rule 6(e)(3)(D) information; or any loss, compromise, or suspected compromise of Rule 6(e)(3)(D) information.

f. (U) **Violations**

i. (U) A Receiving Official who knowingly violates Rule 6(e)(3)(D) by using the disclosed information outside the conduct of his or her official duties, or by failing to adhere to any limitations on the dissemination of such information, may be subject to contempt of court proceedings and to restriction on future receipt of Rule 6(e)(3)(D) information.

ii. (U) A state, local, Indian tribal, or foreign government official who receives Rule 6(e)(3)(D) information, and who knowingly violates these guidelines, may be subject to contempt of court proceedings.

iii. (U) An attorney for the government who knowingly violates Rule 6(e)(3)(D) may be subject to contempt of court proceedings.

g. (U) **Limitation on Unauthorized Disclosures**.

(U) Rule 6(e)(3)(D)(i) provides that Receiving Officials may use disclosed information only to conduct their "official duties subject to any limitation on the unauthorized disclosure of such information." This "limitation on unauthorized disclosures" is understood to encompass applicable statutory, regulatory, and guideline restrictions regarding classification, privacy, or other information protection, as well as any additional restrictions imposed by the federal prosecutor.

(U//FOUO) **Note:** The FGJ-Guidelines do not require that the Receiving Official notify the federal prosecutor of subsequent disclosures, except for consultation for public disclosures and consent for certain disclosures by foreign officials. The Receiving Official is bound by whatever restrictions govern his or her use and disclosure of the information as part of his official duties. (Memo dated 5/15/08, Guidelines for the Disclosure and Use of FGJ Information under Rule 6[e][3][D]).

h. (U//FOUO) **Limitation of Use**

   i. (U//FOUO) Because of the restrictions involved in handling information that is   b2
      obtained by the use of a grand jury subpoena, whenever possible, alternatives to   b7E
      the grand jury subpoena, such as [   ]
      [   ] should be considered as an alternative method of obtaining
      evidence.

   ii. (U) A grand jury subpoena may only be used for purposes of gathering information that is relevant to the grand jury's investigation. Grand jury secrecy continues indefinitely, regardless of whether there is an indictment, unless the material becomes a matter of public record, such as by being introduced at trial.

   iii. (U) Rule 6(e)(3)(D) does not require notice to the court of subsequent dissemination of the information by Receiving Officials.

   iv. (U//FOUO) Disclosure of grand jury material cannot be made within the FBI for unrelated investigations unless a government attorney has determined that such disclosure to a particular investigator is needed to assist that attorney in a specific criminal investigation. The ability of government attorneys to freely share grand jury material with other government attorneys for related or unrelated criminal investigations does not extend to investigators without case specific authorization from the government attorney and notice to the court. Therefore, grand jury material must be restricted when placed into a general system of records that is freely accessible to FBI employees and others with access (e.g., ACS).

   v. (U//FOUO) If a government attorney authorizes the disclosure of grand jury material in the possession of the FBI for use in an unrelated federal criminal matter, such approval should be documented in the grand jury subfile of both the initiated case file and the subsequent case file. That documentation will be in addition to any necessary supplementation to the government attorney's FRCP Rule 6(e) disclosure letter and/or to the internal disclosure list.

vi. (U//FOUO) The USAO should be consulted immediately for precautionary instructions if grand jury material will have application to civil law enforcement functions (e.g., civil RICO or civil forfeiture). There are very limited exceptions that allow government attorneys to use grand jury material or information in civil matters (e.g., civil penalty proceedings concerning banking law violations). These exceptions do not automatically apply to investigative personnel. Therefore, any similar use of grand jury information by the FBI must be approved in advance by the government attorney.

vii. (U//FOUO) Disclosure cannot be made without a court order for use in non-criminal investigations, such as background investigations or name checks.

viii. (U//FOUO) Government personnel who are preparing a response to a Freedom of Information Act or Privacy Act request may properly access grand jury material under the Rule because they are considered to be assisting the grand jury attorney by ensuring against any improper disclosure.

i. (U) **Matters Occurring Before the Grand Jury**

i. (U) **Core Grand Jury Material:** There can be no dissemination of matters occurring before the grand jury unless such dissemination comes within one of the exceptions discussed above. There is no uniform legal definition of what constitutes matters occurring before the grand jury except for what is generally referred to as "core" grand jury material. "Core grand jury material" includes the following: (i) names of targets and witnesses; (ii) grand jury testimony; (iii) grand jury subpoenas; (iv) documents with references to grand jury testimony (including summaries and analyses); (v) documents that clearly reveal the intentions or direction of the grand jury investigation; and (vi) other material that reveals the strategy, direction, testimony, or other proceedings of a grand jury.

ii. (U) **Documents Created Independent of Grand Jury but Obtained by Grand Jury Subpoena:** Rule 6(e) generally prohibits disclosing "matters occurring before the grand jury." The rule, however, does not define that phrase. The issue of whether pre-existing documents fall within that prohibition has never been settled conclusively by the Supreme Court, although many lower courts have discussed it at length. Courts generally agree that this prohibition does not cover all information developed in the course of a grand jury investigation; rather, the secrecy rule applies only to information that would reveal the existence, strategy or direction of the grand jury investigation, the nature of the evidence produced before the grand jury, the views expressed by members of the grand jury, or anything else that actually occurred before the grand jury. In addition, courts have frequently held that Rule 6(e) does not protect documents subpoenaed from the government that are sought by third parties only for the information contained within the document rather than to determine the direction or strategy of the grand jury investigation. Due to developing law on this issue, FBI personnel should consult with the AUSA responsible to determine how to best handle these documents.

iii. (U//FOUO) **Data Extracted from Records Obtained by Grand Jury Subpoena:** Information extracted from business records that was obtained by grand jury subpoena is often used to facilitate investigations. Some of that type of data is, by statute or case law, subject to "the Rule." In other cases, determination of whether data must be considered subject to "the Rule" depends on the case law and local practice in the federal district. Information extracted from grand jury subpoenaed financial records subject to the Right to Financial Privacy Act of 1978 (12 U.S.C. § 3420) must be treated as grand jury material "unless such record has been used in the prosecution of a crime for which the grand jury issued an indictment or presentment...." With the approval of the USAO, information from subpoenaed telephone records may be disclosed for use in unrelated federal criminal investigations in those districts where such material is not considered a "matter occurring before a grand jury." If the USAO approves generally of this procedure, such information may be used in unrelated criminal investigations without authorization from a government attorney in each instance.

j. (U) **Federal Grand Jury Physical Evidence and Statements of Witnesses**

i. (U) Physical evidence provided to the government in response to a grand jury subpoena is subject to the secrecy rule regardless of whether such evidence is presented to the grand jury. Physical evidence provided voluntarily or obtained by means other than grand jury process (such as by a search warrant) is not a grand jury matter regardless of whether such evidence was previously or is thereafter presented to the grand jury.

ii. (U) Statements of witnesses obtained as a result of grand jury process including grand jury subpoena, such as a statement given in lieu of grand jury testimony, are matters occurring before the grand jury irrespective of whether such witnesses testified before the grand jury or are not required to testify. Voluntary statements of witnesses made outside of the grand jury context (not pursuant to any grand jury process including a grand jury subpoena), including statements made outside the grand jury by a witness who is being prepared for grand jury testimony, are not grand jury matters irrespective of whether the witness previously testified or will thereafter testify before the grand jury.

iii. (U) Rule 6(e)(3)(B) requires a federal prosecutor who discloses grand jury material to government investigators and other persons supporting the grand jury investigation to promptly provide the court that impaneled the grand jury the names of the persons to whom such disclosure has been made and to certify that he/she has advised such persons of their obligation of secrecy under the Rule. In order to document the certification required by the Rule, government attorneys often execute and deliver to the court a form, normally referred to as a "Certification" or "Rule 6(e) letter." A copy of this document should be maintained with the grand jury material held in the FBI's custody.

iv. (U//FOUO) **Documentation of Internal Disclosures of Grand Jury Material:** Grand jury material should be kept in such as fashion as to maintain the integrity of the evidence. Upon taking custody of grand jury material, the FBI employee should categorize it in a manner to identify its production source and how it was obtained, to include the identity of a custodian of record for documentary evidence. Practical considerations often require agents assisting government attorneys to seek assistance in the same investigation from others within the FBI. In many districts, support personnel and supervisors of case agents need not be routinely included in the list provided to the court. In lieu of a Rule 6(e) letter from the USAO containing an exhaustive list of names of FBI personnel, an FBI record of additional internal disclosures must be maintained by the case agent in order to establish accountability. Use of this "internal certification" procedure should be authorized by the appropriate USAO. The internal form should record the date of disclosure as well as the identity and position of the recipient. Such internal disclosures may be made only in support of the same investigation in which a federal prosecutor has previously issued a Rule 6(e) letter. In addition, the internal record should reflect that all recipients of grand jury materials were advised of the secrecy requirements of Rule 6(e). Whenever practicable, recipients should be listed on this internal certification prior to disclosure. Local Rule 6(e) customs should govern the internal certification process used.

v. (U//FOUO) **Storage of Grand Jury Material:** The FBI cannot make or allow unauthorized disclosure of grand jury material. Material and records obtained pursuant to the grand jury process are frequently stored in FBI space. FBI personnel should report any unauthorized disclosure to the appropriate government attorney who, in turn, must notify the court. In order to protect against unauthorized disclosure, grand jury material must be secured in the following manner:

1. (U//FOUO) The cover, envelope, or container containing grand jury materials must be marked with the warning: "GRAND JURY MATERIAL - DISSEMINATE ONLY PURSUANT TO RULE 6(e)." No Grand Jury stamp or mark should be affixed to the original material. Agents, analysts and other authorized parties should work from copies of grand jury material whenever possible to ensure the original material retains its integrity.

2. (U//FOUO) Access to grand jury material must be limited to authorized persons (e.g., those assisting an attorney for the government in a specific criminal investigation). All necessary precautions should be taken to protect grand jury material, to include maintaining the material in a secure location when not in use. The material must be appropriately segregated, secured, and safeguarded. Absent chain-of-custody considerations, grand jury material may be maintained in the 1A section of the file. Grand jury material need not be kept in an evidence or bulky exhibit room and may be entrusted to a support services technician (SST) or evidence control technician (ECT). Should grand jury material be entered into a computer database, the data must be marked with the 6(e) warning and maintained within the system in a restricted manner.

3. (U//FOUO) Registered mail or other traceable courier (such as Federal Express) approved by the Chief Security Officer (CSO) must be used to mail or transmit to other Field Offices any documents containing grand jury material. Couriers and other personnel employed in these services will not be aware of the contents of the material transmitted because of the wrapping procedures specified below, and therefore, then do not require a background investigation for this purpose. The names of persons who transport the material need not be placed on a disclosure list, but the receiving office must provide the case agent in the originating office with the names of personnel in the receiving office to whom disclosure is made.

4. (U//FOUO) Grand jury material that is to be mailed or transmitted by traceable courier outside a facility must be enclosed in opaque inner and outer covers. The inner cover must be a sealed wrapper or envelope that contains the addresses of the sender and the addressee, who must be authorized to have access to the grand jury material. The inner cover must be conspicuously marked "Grand Jury Information To Be Opened By Addressee Only." The outer cover must be sealed, addressed, return addressed, and bear no indication that the envelope contains grand jury material. When the size, weight, or nature of the grand jury material precludes the use of envelopes or standard packaging, the material used for packaging or covering must be of sufficient strength and durability to protect the information from unauthorized disclosure or accidental exposure.

5. (U//FOUO) If the government attorney determines that the sensitivity of, or threats to, grand jury material necessitates a more secure transmission method, the material may be transmitted by an express mail service approved for the transmission of national security information or be hand carried by the assigned government attorney or his or her designated representative.

6. (U//FOUO) Grand jury material containing classified national security information must be handled, processed, and stored according to 28 C.F.R.

Part 17. Grand jury material containing other types of sensitive information, such as federal tax return information, witness security information, and other types of highly sensitive information that have more stringent security requirements than that usually required for grand jury material must be stored and protected pursuant to the security regulations governing such information and any special security instructions provided by the organization that originated the information.

7. (U//FOUO) Original documents that are obtained through the grand jury process should be returned to the attorney for the government or, with the government attorney's permission, to the owner if there is no indictment or the prosecution has concluded.

k. (U) **Requests for Subpoenas in Fugitive Investigations**

(U//FOUO) It is generally a misuse of the grand jury to use the grand jury as an investigative aid in the search for a fugitive. Therefore, with the exceptions discussed below, grand jury subpoenas for testimony or records related to the fugitive's whereabouts may not be requested in FBI fugitive investigations.

i. (U//FOUO) Grand jury process may be used to locate a fugitive if the grand jury is interested in hearing the fugitive's testimony. Thus, if the grand jury seeks the testimony of the fugitive in an investigation that the grand jury is indicting, the grand jury may subpoena other witnesses and records in an effort to locate the fugitive witness. However, interest in the fugitive's testimony must not be a pretext. The sole motive for inquiring into the fugitive's location must be the potential value of fugitive's testimony to the grand jury's investigation. A subpoena for the fugitive witness must be approved by the grand jury before seeking to subpoena witnesses or records to locate the fugitive. Further, it is not proper to seek to obtain grand jury testimony from any witness, including a fugitive, concerning an already-returned indictment. Thus, it would not be proper to seek to locate a fugitive for the purpose of having the fugitive testify about matters for which an indictment has already been returned, unless there are additional unindicted defendants to be discovered or additional criminal acts to be investigated through the testimony of the fugitive. Current policy on "target" witnesses must be observed. Grand jury subpoenas for witnesses and records aimed at locating a fugitive witness who is a target of the grand jury investigation should be sought only where a target subpoena for the fugitive has already been approved by the responsible Assistant Attorney General.

ii. (U//FOUO) Use of the grand jury to learn the present location of a fugitive is also proper when the present location is an element of the offense under investigation. On adequate facts, the present location of a fugitive might tend to establish that another person is harboring the fugitive, or has committed misprision, or is an accessory after the fact in the present concealment of the fugitive. However, this justification would likely be viewed as a subterfuge if the suspected harborer or the person potentially guilty of misprision or as an accessory were given immunity in the grand jury in order to compel his/her testimony about the location of the fugitive. With regard to escaped federal prisoner and bond default matters, the present location of a fugitive is not relevant evidence in a grand jury investigation because these offenses address the circumstances of a prior departure from a known location. The fugitive's present location is not a relevant factor as it is in harboring or as it may be in a misprision investigation. Inasmuch as unlawful flight to avoid prosecution cases are, as a rule, not prosecuted and cannot be prosecuted without written authorization from the Attorney General or an Assistant Attorney General, any effort to use the grand jury in the investigation of such cases must be preceded by consultation with the DOJ and by written authorization to prosecute from the Assistant Attorney General in charge of the Criminal Division.

11.9.2. (U) Administrative Subpoena

A. (U) Summary

(U) The Attorney General of the United States is vested with the authority to issue administrative subpoenas under two provisions of the United States Code that have relevance to FBI criminal investigations, 21 U.S.C. § 876 and 18 U.S.C. § 3486. The FBI has no inherent authority to issue administrative subpoenas but relies on delegated authority from the Attorney General. The use of administrative subpoenas is limited to three categories of investigations—drug program investigations, child sexual exploitation and abuse investigations, and health care fraud investigations—and may not be used for any other purpose. The delegated authority varies depending on the federal violation being investigated. The type of information that can be obtained using an administrative subpoena is also limited by law or by policy of the Attorney General.

(U//FOUO) **Note:** Within the FBI, the authority to issue administrative subpoenas is limited to those positions holding the delegated authority from the Attorney General; that authority may not be redelegated.

b2
b7E

B. (U) Legal Authority and Delegation

1. (U) **Investigations involving the sale, transfer, manufacture or importation of unlawful drugs**

    (U) **Authority:** 21 U.S.C. § 876 and DOJ Regulation at 28 C.F.R. App to Pt. 0, Subpt. R § 4.

    (U) **May be issued to:** Any individual or business holding records relevant to the drug investigation.

    (U) **Records to be obtained:** Any records relevant to the investigation.

    (U//FOUO) **Delegated authority to issue:** By DOJ regulation, the Attorney General's delegation includes SACs, ASACs, SSRAs and "those FBI Special Agent Squad

Supervisors who have management responsibilities over Organized Crime/Drug Program investigations."

(U//FOUO) [   ]   b2
b7E

(U//FOUO) **Limitations:** [   ]   b2
b7E

[   ] The Right to Financial Privacy Act limitations described in paragraph D of this section apply. If addressed to a provider of "electronic communication service" or a "remote computing service," provisions in the Electronic Communication Privacy Act (ECPA) govern, as discussed in paragraph D of this section.

2. (U) **Investigations involving the sexual exploitation or abuse of children**

(U) **Authority:** 18 U.S.C. § 3486(a) and Attorney General Order 2718-2004.

(U) **May be issued to:** A "provider of an electronic communication service" or a "remote computer service" (both terms defined in Section 11.9.2.D.2.b, below) and only for the production of basic subscriber or customer information. The subpoena may require production as soon as possible but in no event less than 24 hours after service of the subpoena.

(U) **Records to be obtained:** [   ]   b2
b7E

(U//FOUO) **Delegated authority to issue:** [   ]   b2
b7E

(U//FOUO) **Limitations:** By law, these administrative subpoenas may only be issued in cases that involve a violation of 18 U.S.C. §§ 1201, 2241(c), 2242, 2243, 2251, 2251A, 2252, 2252A, 2260, 2421, 2422, or 2423 in which the victim has not attained the age of 18 years. Under the Attorney General's delegation, an administrative subpoena in these investigations may be issued only to "providers of electronic communication services" or to "remote computing services" to obtain the information listed above. These administrative subpoenas may not be issued to any other person or entity or to obtain any other information, including the content of communications.

b2
b7E

3. (U) Investigations involving Federal Health Care Fraud Offenses

(U) **Authority:** 18 U.S.C. § 3486(a)

(U) **Records to be obtained:** Records relevant to an investigation relating to a "federal health care offense." Federal health care offense is defined in 18 U.S.C. § 24

(U) **May be issued to:** Any public or private entity or individual with records relevant to the federal health care offense. (**Note:** These are referred to in guidance issued by the Attorney General as "investigative demands.")

(U//FOUO) **Delegated authority to issue:** There is no delegation to the FBI. Delegated to personnel within DOJ's Criminal Division and to United States Attorneys, who may redelegate the authority to Assistant United States Attorneys.

(U) **Limitations:** The Right to Financial Privacy Act (RFPA) limitations described in paragraph D of this section apply. The provisions in ECPA govern, as discussed in paragraph D of this section, if the request for records is addressed to a "provider of electronic communication service" or a "remote computing service." The subpoena may not require the production of records at a place more than 500 miles from the place the subpoena is served.

b2
b7E

(U) **Restriction on individual health care information:** Pursuant to 18 U.S.C. § 3486, health information about an individual acquired through an authorized investigative demand may not be used in, or disclosed to any person for use in, any administrative, civil, or criminal action against that individual unless the action or investigation arises from and is directly related to receipt of health care, payment for health care, or action involving a fraudulent claim related to health care.

(U//FOUO)

b2
b7E

C. (U) **Approval Requirements**

(U//FOUO) Use of an administrative subpoena requires SSA approval. The SSA may issue the administrative subpoena if the authority has been so delegated. Further review and approval may be required depending on the delegation. Review by the CDC is appropriate if legal questions arise in preparing and issuing the subpoena.

(U//FOUO) **Note:** An individual designated by proper authority to serve in an "acting" status in one of the positions with delegated authority may sign and issue an administrative subpoena. The "acting" status should be documented in an appropriate Field Office administrative file and noted in the case file. For example, if the ASAC with authority to sign is away on leave or temporary duty and another individual has been designated by the SAC to serve as "acting" ASAC, that individual has authority to issue the administrative subpoena.

154

A relief supervisor is not considered to be in an "acting" status for purposes of issuing an administrative subpoena.

D. (U) Limitations on Use of Administrative Subpoenas

1. (U) Financial Privacy Limitations

   a. (U) **Obtaining records from a financial institution.** "Financial records" are those records that pertain to a customer's relationship with a financial institution. The term "financial institution" is broadly defined as a bank, savings bank, card issuer, industrial loan company, trust company, savings association, building and loan or homestead association, credit union, or consumer finance institution, located in any state, territory, or the District of Columbia. See 12 U.S.C. § 3401. [**Note:** The scope of the RFPA's definition of financial institution for this purpose, which limits the restrictions the RFPA places on federal law enforcement in using an administrative subpoena, is narrower than the definition of financial institution that is used in connection with NSLs. For that purpose, the RFPA refers to the broader definition found in the Bank Secrecy Act (BSA). Among the entities included in the BSA definition are money transmitting businesses, car dealers, travel agencies, and persons involved in real estate closings. See 12 U.S.C. § 3414(d) and 31 U.S.C. § 5312.(a)(2) and (c)(1).] When seeking financial records from a financial institution, the FBI must send a certificate of compliance required by 12 U.S.C. § 3403 to the financial institution. The certificate must indicate, among other things, that notice has been provided by the FBI to the individual customer whose financial records are to be obtained. The content of the notice is set out in 12 U.S.C. § 3405. A court order may be obtained that allows for delayed notice pursuant to 12 U.S.C. § 3409. Notice is not required if the administrative subpoena is issued to obtain the financial records of a corporation or for records not pertaining to a customer. Notice is also not required if the administrative subpoena seeks only basic account information, defined as name, address, type of account, and account number. See 12 U.S.C. § 3413(g).

   b. (U) **Obtaining records from a Credit Bureau.** A credit bureau or consumer reporting agency may only provide name, address, former addresses, place of employment and former place of employment in response to an administrative subpoena. 15 U.S.C. § 1681f. A credit bureau or consumer reporting agency may not release financial information in a credit report or consumer report, or the names and locations of financial institutions at which the consumer has accounts pursuant to an administrative subpoena. A court order, a grand jury subpoena, or, in an appropriate case, a national security letter may be used to obtain this information. 15 U.S.C. § 1681b. Notice of disclosure will be provided by the credit bureau or consumer reporting agency to the consumer if the consumer requests this information.

2. (U) Electronic Communication Privacy Act

   a. (U) **Use of an Administrative Subpoena.** The ability to gather subscriber information and the content of electronic communications using an administrative subpoena is governed by ECPA. In cases involving the sexual exploitation or abuse of children, only basic subscriber or customer information may be obtained with an administrative subpoena under the terms of the Attorney General's delegation, as described above. No content information may be obtained. In drug and health care fraud investigations, an administrative subpoena may be used to obtain basic subscriber or customer information and certain stored communications, under limited circumstances, from entities that provide electronic communication services to the public.

b. (U) **Definitions.** ECPA applies to two types of entities that provide electronic communications to the public. The term "provider of electronic communication services" is defined in 18 U.S.C. § 2510(15) as "any service that provides the user thereof the ability to send or receive wire or electronic communications." The term "remote computing services" is defined in 18 U.S.C. § 2711(12) as the "provision to the public of computer storage or processing services by means of an electronic communication system."

c. (U) **Subscriber information.**

b2
b7E

d. (U) **Records or other information pertaining to a subscriber.**

b2
b7E

e. (U) **Content.** Content is the actual substance of files stored in an account, including the subject line of an e-mail.

(1) (U) Unopened e-mail held in storage for 180 days or less may not be obtained using an administrative subpoena. A search warrant is required.

(2) (U) Unopened e-mail that has been held in electronic storage for more than 180 days may be obtained with an administrative subpoena. (In the Ninth Circuit, the opened e-mail and un-opened e-mail must have been in storage for 180 days before it can be obtained with an administrative subpoena. See Theofel v. Farey-Jones, 359 F.3d 1066.) The government must provide notice to the subscriber or customer prior to obtaining such content. A limited exception to the notice requirement is provided in 18 U.S.C. § 2705.

(3) (U) E-mail that has been opened and the content of other electronically stored files held in storage by an entity that provides storage services to the public (i.e., a remote computing service, as defined in 18 U.S.C. § 2711), may be obtained using an administrative subpoena with notice to the customer or subscriber, unless notice is delayed in accordance with 18 U.S.C. § 2705.

(4) (U) E-mail that has been opened and the content of other electronically stored files held in storage by an entity that does not provide electronic communication services to the public, such as that on the internal network of a business, may be obtained using an administrative subpoena. Notice to the individual is not required because this demand is not restricted by ECPA.

3. (U//FOUO) **Members of the Media**

(U//FOUO) An administrative subpoena directed to a provider of electronic communication services or any other entity seeking to obtain local and long distance connection records, or records of session times of calls, made by a member of the news media may only be issued with the specific approval of the Attorney General. Requests for this approval should be reviewed by the CDC and coordinated with an Assistant United States Attorney (AUSA). The request must provide justification for issuance of the subpoena consistent with the Department of Justice policies set forth in 28 C.F.R. § 50.10. Guidance on this policy may be obtained from the Investigative Law Unit and/or the Privacy and Civil Liberties Unit, OGC.

E. (U//FOUO) **Compliance/Monitoring**

1. (U) **Limits on use.**

b2
b7E

2. (U//FOUO) **Overproduction.**

b2
b7E

3. (U//FOUO) **Factors for compliance.** The following factors should be considered to ensure compliance with applicable laws and regulations that govern the FBI's use of administrative subpoenas:

a. (U//FOUO) The administrative subpoena must relate to a type of investigation for which the subpoena is authorized;

b. (U//FOUO) The administrative subpoena must be directed to a recipient to whom an administrative subpoena is authorized;

c. (U//FOUO) The administrative subpoena may request only records that are authorized under the pertinent law;

d. (U//FOUO) The administrative subpoena must be approved by an authorized official;

e. (U//FOUO) The administrative subpoena must be uploaded into the Automated Case Support (ACS) system to the Subpoena ("SBP") subfile of the substantive case file for record purposes;

f. (U//FOUO) The return of service information must be completed on the back of the original administrative subpoena;

g. (U//FOUO) The original administrative subpoena and completed return of service must be maintained in a "SBP" subfile of the substantive investigation; and

h. (U//FOUO) The records provided in response to the administrative subpoena must be reviewed to ensure that the FBI is authorized to collect the records provided. If an over-production has occurred, steps must be taken to correct the error.

11.9.3.   (U) National Security Letter

A. (U) **Legal Authority**

(U) 15 U.S.C. §§ 1681u, 1681v; 18 U.S.C. § 2709;

(U) 12 U.S.C. § 3414(a) (5) (A); 50 U.S.C. § 436;

(U) AGG-Dom, Part V

(U) A National Security Letter (NSL) may be used only to request:

1. (U) **Financial Records:** The Right to Financial Privacy Act (RFPA), 12 U.S.C. § 3414(a)(5);

2. (U) **Identity of Financial Institutions:** Fair Credit Reporting Act (FCRA), 15 U.S.C. § 1681u(a);

3. (U) **Consumer Identifying Information:** FCRA, 15 U.S.C. § 1681u(b);

4. (U) **Identity of Financial Institutions and Consumer Identifying Information:** FCRA, 15 U.S.C. §§ 1681u(a) & (b);

5. (U) **Full Credit Reports in International Terrorism Investigations:** FCRA, 15 U.S.C. § 1681v; and

6. (U) **Telephone Subscriber Information, Toll Billing Records, Electronic Communication Subscriber Information, and Electronic Communication Transactional Records:** Electronic Communications Privacy Act (ECPA), 18 U.S.C. § 2709.

B. (U) **Definition of Method**

(U) A National Security Letter is an administrative demand for documents or records that can be made by the FBI during a predicated investigation relevant to a threat to the national security. Sample NSLs are available.

C. (U//FOUO) **Approval Requirements**

(U//FOUO) A request for an NSL has two parts. One is the NSL itself, and one is the EC approving the issuance of the NSL. The authority to sign NSLs has been delegated to the

Deputy Director, Executive Assistant Director and Assistant EAD for the National Security Branch; Assistant Directors and all DADs for CT/CD/Cyber; General Counsel; Deputy General Counsel for the National Security Law Branch; Assistant Directors in Charge in NY, DC, and LA; and all SACs.

(U//FOUO) In addition to being signed by a the statutorily-required approver, every NSL must be reviewed and approved by a CDC, ADC or attorney acting in that capacity, or an NSLB attorney.

(U)

b2
b7E

(U//FOUO)

b2
b7E

(U//FOUO)

b2
b7E

(U//FOUO)

b2
b7E

(U//FOUO)

b2
b7E

b2
b7E

D. (U) Duration of Approval

b2
b7E

E. (U//FOUO) Specific Procedures

(U//FOUO)

b2
b7E

(U//FOUO)

b2
b7E

(U//FOUO)

b2
b7E

- (U//FOUO)

b2
b7E

- (U//FOUO)

b2
b7E

- (U//FOUO)

b2
b7E

- (U//FOUO)

b2
b7E

(U//FOUO)

b2
b7E

b2
b7E

b2
b7E

(U//FOUO)

1. (U//FOUO) **Cover EC**

    (U//FOUO)

    b2
    b7E

    a. (U//FOUO)

    b. (U//FOUO)

    c. (U//FOUO)

    d. (U//FOUO)

    b2
    b7E

    e. (U//FOUO)

    f. (U//FOUO)

    g. (U//FOUO)

    h. (U//FOUO)

    i. (U//FOUO)

    j. (U//FOUO)

k. (U//FOUO[   ] b2
    [   ] b7E

l. (U//FOUO)[   ]
    [   ]
    [   ]

(U//FOUO[   ] b2
[   ] b7E

2. (U) **Copy of NSL**

    (U//FOUO) A copy of the signed NSL must be retained in the investigative case file and uploaded under the appropriate NSL document type in ACS. Documented proof of service of NSL letters must be maintained in the case file.

3. (U//FOUO) **Second Generation Information**

    (U//FOUO[   ]

    [   ] b2
                                                               b7E

4. (U//FOUO) **Emergency Circumstances**

    (U//FOUO) ECPA protects subscriber or transactional information regarding communications from disclosure by providers of telephone or other electronic communication services. Generally, an NSL, grand jury subpoena, or other forms of legal process must be used to compel the communication service provider to disclose subscriber or transactional information. In emergency circumstances, however, if the provider in good faith believes that a delay in disclosure could pose a danger of death or serious bodily injury, the provider may voluntarily disclose information to the FBI. As a matter of FBI policy, when there is a danger of death or serious bodily injury that does not permit the proper processing of an NSL, if approved by an ASAC, a letter to the provider citing 18 U.S.C. § 2702 may be used to request emergency disclosure. If time does not permit the issuance of an emergency letter citing 18 U.S.C. § 2702, an oral request to the provider may be made, but the oral request must be followed-up with a letter as described herein.

    (U//FOUO)[   ]

    [   ] b2
                                                               b7E

162

b2
b7E

(U//FOUO)

b2
b7E

(U//FOUO)

b2
b7E

F. (U//FOUO) **Notice and Reporting Requirements**

(U//FOUO) The National Security Law Branch at FBIHQ is required to report information about NSL usage to Congress. The data necessary for Congressional reporting is automatically recorded if the NSL is created in the NSL Subsystem (FISAMS). If the NSL is created outside the system, the EC must include all information necessary for NSLB accurately to report NSL statistics. The EC must break down the number of targeted phone numbers/e-mail accounts/financial accounts that are addressed to each and every NSL recipient. Therefore, if there are three targets, ten accounts, and six recipients of an NSL, the EC must state how many accounts are the subject of the NSL as to Recipient 1, Recipient 2, etc. It is not sufficient to only indicate that there are ten accounts and six recipients.

(U//FOUO) In addition, the FBI must report the United States person status of the subject of all NSL requests (as opposed to the target of the investigation to which the NSL is relevant), other than those seeking subscriber information. While the subject is often the target of the investigation, that is not always the case. The EC must reflect the United States person status of the subject of the request – the person whose information the FBI is seeking. If the NSL is seeking information about more than one person, the EC must reflect the United States person status of each of those persons. (See the form ECs, which make clear that the United States person status applies to the target of the request for information.)

(U//FOUO) Finally, to ensure accurate reporting, the EC must accurately state the type of information that is being sought. NSLs for toll billing records or transactional records will include subscriber information. The EC need only state that the request is for toll billing records or transactional records, and the reporting paragraph should state that toll billing or transactional records are being sought for x number of accounts, and, if multiple recipients, from each of recipients #1, #2, etc.

G. (U//FOUO) **Receipt of NSL Information**

(U//FOUO

b2
b7E

b2
b7E

(U//FOUO)

b2
b7E

(U//FOUO)

b2
b7E

(U//FOUO)

b2
b7E

H. (U//FOUO) **Dissemination of NSL material**

(U//FOUO) Subject to certain statutory limitations, information obtained through the use of an NSL may be disseminated according to general dissemination standards in the AGG-Dom. ECPA (telephone and electronic communications records) and the RFPA (financial records) permit dissemination if consistent with the AGG-Dom and if the information is clearly relevant to the responsibilities of the recipient agency. FCRA, 15 U.S.C. § 1681u, permits dissemination to other federal agencies as may be necessary for the approval or conduct of a foreign counterintelligence investigation. FCRA imposes no special rules for dissemination of full credit reports.

(U//FOUO) the NSLs themselves are not classified, nor is the material received in return.

b2
b7E

b2
b7E

I. (U) **Payment for NSL-Derived Information**

(U//FOUO) Because there is no legal obligation for the FBI to compensate recipients of NSLs issued pursuant to ECPA, 18 U.S.C. § 2709 (toll billing records information, subscriber, electronic communication transactional records) or FCRA, 15 U.S.C. § 1681v, (full credit reports in international terrorism cases), there should not be payment in connection with those NSLs. See EC, 319X-HQ-A1487720-OGC, serial 222, for a form letter to be sent in response to demands for payment for these types of NSLs.

(U) Compensation is legally required for NSLs served to obtain financial information pursuant to RFPA, 12 U.S.C. § 3414(a)(5), and credit information pursuant to FCRA, 15 U.S.C. § 1681u. Under 12 C.F.R. § 219.3, Appendix A, a fee schedule has been adopted under which photocopying is reimbursable at $.25 per page and searching is reimbursable at $11 per hour for clerical staff. Regulations governing a payment schedule for FCRA, 15 U.S.C. § 1681u, NSLs has not been promulgated.

11.9.4. (U) Business Record Under FISA

A. (U) **Legal Authority**

(U) 50 U.S.C. §§ 1861-63

B. (U) **Definition of Method**

(U) A FISA order for business records is an order for a third party to produce documents, records and other tangible information relevant to a predicated national security investigation. FISA Business Record Orders may not be used to obtain information during a positive foreign intelligence case if the material sought relates to a United States person. There is no "FISA-derived" impediment to the use of documents obtained pursuant to such orders.

C. (U//FOUO) **Approval Requirements**

b2
b7E

D. (U) **Duration of Approval**

(U) Duration is established by the court order.

E. (U) **Notice and Reporting Requirements**

(U) There are no special notice or reporting requirements.

F. (U) Compliance Requirements

(U) The case agent who receives production of documents pursuant to a FISA business records order must do the following:

1. (U//FOUO) Handle the production as required by the Standard Minimization Procedures Adopted for Business Record Orders

    b2
    b7E

2. (U) Whether or not required by paragraph 1, prior to uploading the documents or data received into FBI databases, review the documents produced to determine whether they are responsive to the order.

    a. (U//FOUO) If the producing party has mistakenly provided material that is entirely non-responsive (e.g., the producing party inverted numbers on an account and produced entirely irrelevant and non-responsive material), the case agent must sequester the material and discuss with the CDC or NSLB the appropriate way to return the unresponsive material to the producing party and obtain the responsive material.

    b. (U//FOUO) If the producing party has produced responsive material and material that is beyond the parameters of the order issued by the FISC (e.g., the FISC ordered production of one month's records and the party produced records for 6 weeks), the case agent must determine whether the material produced that is outside the parameters of the FISC order is subject to statutory protection (e.g., records that are subject to the Right to Financial Privacy Act, the Buckley Amendments, the Electronic Communications Privacy Act, Fair Credit Reporting Act).

        i. (U//FOUO) If the overproduced material is subject to statutory protection, then the overproduced material must be treated like overproduction is treated in the context of a national security letter.

        ii. (U//FOUO) If the overproduced material is not subject to statutory protection, then it may be uploaded. In determining whether to upload the overproduced material, the case agent should consider the extent to which the overproduction includes non-public information regarding United States persons who are not the subject of a national security investigation; the sensitivity of the information contained within the overproduction; and the burdensomeness of separating the overproduced material from the responsive material.

11.10. (U) Investigative Method: Accessing stored wire and electronic communications and transactional records in conformity with chapter 121 of title 18, United States Code

11.10.1. (U) Summary

(U//FOUO) FBI employees may acquire the contents of stored wire or electronic communications and associated transactional records—including basic subscriber information—as provided in 18 U.S.C. §§ 2701-2712. Requests for voluntary disclosure under the emergency authority of 18 U.S.C. § 2702 require prior approval from the Field Office ASAC or FBIHQ Section Chief when appropriate.

(U//FOUO) **Application:** This investigative method may be used during national security investigations and criminal investigations as authorized by statute. This method may not be used for assistance to other agencies, unless relevant to an already open predicated investigation. This method cannot be used to collect positive foreign intelligence. Additionally, this method cannot be used during an assessment.

A. (U) **Stored Data:** The Electronic Communications Privacy Act (ECPA)—18 U.S.C. §§ 2701-2712—governs the disclosure of two broad categories of information: (i) the contents of wire or electronic communications held in "electronic storage" by providers of "electronic communication service" or contents held by those who provide "remote computing service" to the public; and (ii) records or other information pertaining to a subscriber to or customer of such services. The category of "records or other information" can be subdivided further into subscriber records (listed in 18 U.S.C. § 2703[c][2]) and stored traffic data or other records.

   (U) Records covered by ECPA include all records that are related to the subscriber, including buddy lists, "friend" lists (MySpace), and virtual property owned (Second Life). These other sorts of records are not subscriber records and cannot be obtained by a subpoena under 18 U.S.C. § 2703(c)(2) or an NSL under 18 U.S.C. § 2709.

B. (U) **Legal Process:** The legal process for obtaining disclosure will vary depending on the type of information sought and whether the information is being voluntarily provided under 18 U.S.C. § 2702 (e.g., with consent or when emergency circumstances require disclosure) or the provider is being compelled to provide the information under 18 U.S.C. § 2703, as outlined below.

C. (U) Contents held in "electronic storage" by a provider of "electronic communication service" for 180 days or less can only be obtained with a search warrant based on probable cause. Accordingly, such records may only be obtained during a full investigation.

   (U) Contents held by those who provide "remote computing service" to the public and contents held in "electronic storage" for more than 180 days by an "electronic communication service" provider can be obtained with: a warrant; a subpoena; or an order issued by a court under 18 U.S.C. § 2703(d) when prior notice has been provided to the customer or subscriber (unless the court has authorized delayed notice).

   (U) Title 18 United States Code Section 2705 establishes the standard to delay notice for an initial period of up to 90 days. Records or other information pertaining to a subscriber to or customer of such services, including basic subscriber information can be obtained with a search warrant or an 18 U.S.C. § 2703(d) order without notice.

D. (U) Basic subscriber information, as described in 18 U.S.C. § 2703(c)(2), can be compelled by a grand jury or administrative subpoena without notice.

E. (U) **Preservation of Stored Data:** The government is authorized under 18 U.S.C. § 2703(f) to direct a provider to preserve records or other information (stored records or communications) in its possession for 90 days (which may be extended for an additional 90-days) pending issuance of applicable legal process for disclosure. To make a preservation request, the FBI must believe that the records will subsequently be sought by appropriate legal process.

F. (U) **Cost reimbursement:** Title 18 United States Code Section 2706 requires the government to reimburse for costs incurred in providing the contents of communications, records, or other information obtained under 18 U.S.C. §§ 2702, 2703, or 2704, except that reimbursement is not required for records or other information maintained by a communications common carrier that relate to telephone toll records and telephone listings obtained under 18 U.S.C. § 2703. In essence, the government does not have to reimburse for the cost of producing records that the provider maintains in the ordinary course of its business.

11.10.2. (U) Legal Authority

(U) 18 U.S.C. §§ 2701-2712

(U) AGG-Dom, Part V.9

(U) ECPA—18 U.S.C. §§ 2701-2712— creates statutory privacy rights for the contents of communications in "electronic storage" and records or other information pertaining to a subscriber to or customer of an "electronic communication service" and a "remote computing service." The statutory protections protect the privacy of an individual's electronic data contained in a networked account—that may otherwise fall outside the scope of the protections afforded by the Fourth Amendment—when such account or its service is owned or managed by a third-party provider.

(U) ECPA generally: (i) prohibits access to the contents of wire or electronic communications while in "electronic storage" unless authorized (18 U.S.C. § 2701); (ii) prohibits a provider of service to the public from disclosing the contents of wire or electronic communications while held in "electronic storage," and divulging to the government any information pertaining to a subscriber to or customer of such service unless authorized (18 U.S.C. § 2702); and (iii) authorizes the government to compel disclosure from a provider of stored contents of a wire or electronic communication and records or other information pertaining to a subscriber to or customer (18 U.S.C. § 2703). ECPA provides for reimbursement of costs incurred in providing the information acquired.

11.10.3. (U) Definition of Investigative Method

A. (U) **Definitions:**

(U) **Electronic Storage:** is "any temporary, intermediate storage of a wire or electronic communication incidental to the electronic transmission thereof," or "any storage of such communication by an electronic communication service for purposes of backup protection of such communication." 18 U.S.C. § 2510(17). In short, "electronic storage" refers only to temporary storage, made in the course of transmission, by a provider of an electronic communication service.

(U) **Remote Computing Service (RCS):** is the "provision to the public of computer storage or processing services by means of an electronic communications system." 18 U.S.C. § 2711(2). In essence, a remote computing service is an off-site computer that stores or processes data for a customer.

(U) **Electronic Communications System:** is "any wire, radio, electromagnetic; photooptical or photoelectronic facilities for the transmission of wire or electronic communications, and any computer facilities or related electronic equipment for the electronic storage of such communications." 18 U.S.C. § 2510(14).

(U) **Electronic Communication Service (ECS):** is "any service that provides to users thereof the ability to send or receive wire or electronic communications." 18 U.S.C. § 2510(15). For example, telephone companies and electronic mail companies generally act as providers of electronic communication services.

(U) ECPA authorities can be divided into two categories: (i) compelled disclosure—legal process to compel providers to disclose the contents of stored wire or electronic communications (including e-mail and voice mail—opened and unopened) and other information such as account records and basic subscriber information; and (ii) voluntary disclosure of such information from service providers. Each of these authorities is discussed below.

B. (U) **Compelled Disclosure:**

1. (U) Title 18 United States Code Section 2703 lists five types of legal process that the government can use to compel a provider to disclose certain kinds of information. The five mechanisms, in descending order of required threshold showing are as follows:

   - (U) Search warrant;
   - (U) 18 U.S.C. § 2703(d) court order with prior notice to the subscriber or customer;
   - (U) 18 U.S.C. § 2703(d) court order without prior notice to the subscriber or customer;
   - (U) Subpoena with prior notice to the subscriber or customer; and
   - (U) Subpoena without prior notice to the subscriber or customer.

169

b2
b7E

2. (U//FOUO) **Notice—Orders Not to Disclose the Existence of a Warrant, Subpoena, or Court Order:** FBI employees may obtain a court order directing network service providers not to disclose the existence of compelled process if the government has no legal duty to notify the customer or subscriber of the process. If an 18 U.S.C. § 2703(d) order or 18 U.S.C. § 2703(a) warrant is being used, a request for a non-disclosure order can be included in the application and proposed order or warrant. If a subpoena is being used to obtain the information, a separate application to a court for a non-disclosure order must be made.

3. (U) **Legal Standard:** A court may order an electronic communications service provider or remote computing service not to disclose the existence of a warrant, subpoena, or court order for such period as the court deems appropriate. The court must enter such an order if it determines that there is reason to believe that notification of the existence of the warrant, subpoena, or court order will result in:

   - (U) Endangering the life or physical safety of an individual;

   - (U) Flight from prosecution;

   - (U) Destruction of or tampering with evidence;

   - (U) Intimidation of potential witnesses; or

   - (U) Otherwise seriously jeopardizing an investigation or unduly delaying a trial. 18 U.S.C. § 2705(b).

4. (U) **Search Warrant:** Investigators can obtain the full contents of a network account with a search warrant. ECPA does not require the government to notify the customer or subscriber when it obtains information from a provider using a search warrant. Warrants issued under 18 U.S.C. § 2703 must comply with either FRCP Rule 41 or an equivalent state warrant. However, all warrants issued pursuant to 18 U.S.C. § 2703 do not require personal service; those warrants issued by a federal court have nationwide jurisdiction (see below); and the warrants may only be served on an electronic communication service or a remote computing service. FRCP Rule 41 also poses the additional requirement on these warrants that a copy of the warrant be left with the provider, and a return and inventory be made.

   (U) Under 18 U.S.C. § 2703(a), with a search warrant issued based on probable cause pursuant to FRCP Rule 41 or an equivalent state warrant, the government may obtain:

   a. (U) "The contents of a wire or electronic communication, that is in electronic storage in an electronic communications system for one hundred and eighty days or less," and

   b. (U) Everything that can be obtained using a 18 U.S.C. § 2703(d) court order with notice.

   (U) In other words, every record and all of the stored contents of an account—including opened and unopened e-mail/voice mail— can be compelled by a search warrant based on probable cause pursuant to FRCP Rule 41. Moreover, because the warrant is issued by a neutral magistrate based on probable cause, obtaining a search warrant effectively insulates the process from challenge under the Fourth Amendment.

(U) **Nationwide Scope:** Search warrants under 18 U.S.C. § 2703(a) may be issued by a federal "court with jurisdiction over the offense under investigation," and may be executed outside the district of the issuing court for material responsive to the warrant. State courts may also issue warrants under 18 U.S.C. § 2703(a), but the statute does not give these warrants effect outside the issuing court's territorial jurisdiction. As with a typical FRCP Rule 41 warrant, investigators must draft an affidavit and a proposed warrant that complies with FRCP Rule 41.

(U) **Service of Process:** Title 18 United States Code Section 2703(a) search warrants are obtained just like any other FRCP Rule 41 search warrant but are typically served on the provider and compel the provider to find and produce the information described in the warrant. ECPA expressly states that the presence of an officer is not required for service or execution of a search warrant issued pursuant to 18 U.S.C. § 2703(a).

5. (U) **Court Order with Prior Notice to the Subscriber or Customer:** Investigators can obtain everything in a network account except for unopened e-mail or voice-mail stored with a provider for 180 days or less using a 18 U.S.C. § 2703(d) court order with prior notice to the subscriber unless they have obtained authority for delayed notice pursuant to 18 U.S.C. § 2705. ECPA distinguishes between the contents of communications that are in "Electronic storage" (e.g., unopened e-mail) for less than 180 days, and those that have been in "Electronic storage" for longer or that are no longer in "Electronic storage" (e.g., opened e-mail).

(U) FBI employees who obtain a court order under 18 U.S.C. § 2703(d), and either give prior notice to the subscriber or comply with the delayed notice provisions of 18 U.S.C. § 2705(a), may obtain:

   a. (U) "The contents of a wire or electronic communication that has been in electronic storage in an electronic communications system for more than one hundred and eighty days." 18 U.S.C. § 2703(a).

   b. (U) "The contents of any wire or electronic communication" held by a provider of remote computing service "on behalf of . . . a subscriber or customer of such remote computing service," 18 U.S.C. §§ 2703(b)(1)(B)(ii), 2703 (b)(2); and

   c. (U) everything that can be obtained using a 18 U.S.C. § 2703(d) court order without notice.

b2
b7E

b2
b7E

b2
b7E

(U) **Legal Standard:** To order delayed notice, the court must find that "there is reason to believe that notification of the existence of the court order may . . . endanger[] the life or physical safety of an individual; [lead to] flight from prosecution; [lead to] destruction of or tampering with evidence; [lead to] intimidation of potential witnesses; or . . . otherwise seriously jeopardiz[e] an investigation or unduly delay[ ] a trial." 18 U.S.C. §§ 2705(a)(1)(A) and 2705(a)(2). The applicant must satisfy this standard anew each time an extension of the delayed notice is sought.

(U) **Nationwide Scope:** Federal court orders under 18 U.S.C. § 2703(d) have effect outside the district of the issuing court. Title 18 United States Code Section 2703(d) orders may compel providers to disclose information even if the information is stored outside the district of the issuing court. See 18 U.S.C. § 2703(d) ("any court that is a court of competent jurisdiction" may issue a 18 U.S.C. § 2703[d] order); 18 U.S.C. § 2711(3) (court of competent jurisdiction includes any federal court having jurisdiction over the offense being investigated without geographic limitation).

(U) Title 18 United States Code Section 2703(d) orders may also be issued by state courts. See 18 U.S.C. §§ 2711(3); 3127(2)(B). Title 18 United States Code Section 2703(d) orders issued by state courts, however, do not have effect outside the jurisdiction of the issuing state. See 18 U.S.C. §§ 2711(3).

6. (U) **Court Order without Prior Notice to the Subscriber or Customer:** FBI employees need an 18 U.S.C. § 2703(d) court order to obtain most account logs and most transactional records.

(U) A court order under 18 U.S.C. § 2703(d) may compel disclosure of:

a. (U) All "record(s) or other information pertaining to a subscriber to or customer of such service (not including the contents of communications [held by providers of electronic communications service and remote computing service])," and

b. (U) Basic subscriber information that can be obtained using a subpoena without notice. 18 U.S.C. § 2703(c)(1).

(U) **Types of Transactional Records:** The broad category of transactional records includes all records held by a service provider that pertain to the subscriber beyond the specific records listed in 2703(c)(1)

b2
b7E

(U//FOUO)

b2
b7E

c. (U) **Cell site and Sector information:** Cell site and sector information is considered "a record or other information pertaining to a subscriber" and therefore, production of historical and prospective cell site and sector information may be compelled by a court order under 18 U.S.C. § 2703(d). Requests made pursuant to 18 U.S.C. § 2703(d) for disclosure of prospective cell site and sector information—which is delivered to law enforcement under Communications Assistance for Law Enforcement Act (CALEA) at the beginning and end of calls— must be combined with an application for pen register/trap and trace device. Some judicial districts will require a showing of probable cause before authorizing the disclosure of prospective cell site and sector information.

d.

b2
b7E

(U//FOUO)

b2
b7E

(U)

b2
b7E

(U)

b2
b7E

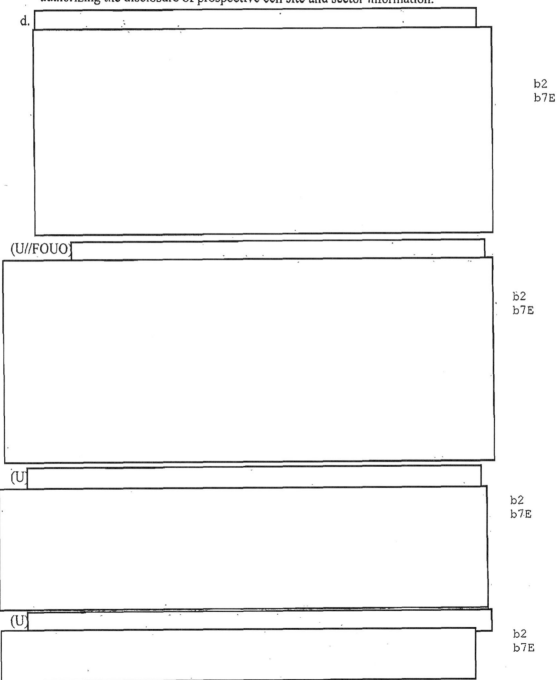

(U) **Legal Standard:** A court order under 18 U.S.C. § 2703(d) is known as an "articulable facts" court order or simply a "d" order. "This section imposes an intermediate standard to protect on-line transactional records. It is a standard higher than a subpoena, but not a probable cause warrant. The intent of raising the standard for access to transactional data is to guard against "fishing expeditions" by law enforcement." (See H.R. Rep. No. 102-827, at 31 (1994), reprinted in 1994 U.S.C.C.A.N. 3489.)

(U) The FBI must state sufficient specific and articulable facts for the court to find that there are reasonable grounds to believe that the contents of a wire or electronic communication, or the records or other information sought, are relevant and material to an ongoing criminal investigation.

b2
b7E

7. (U) **Subpoena with Prior Notice to the Subscriber or Customer:** Investigators can subpoena opened e-mail from a provider if they either give prior notice to the subscriber or comply with the delayed notice provisions of 18 U.S.C. § 2705(a)—which requires a written certification by the SAC or ASAC that there is reason to believe that notification of the existence of the subpoena may have an adverse result.

(U) FBI employees who obtain a subpoena and either give prior notice to the subscriber or comply with the delayed notice provisions of 18 U.S.C. § 2705(a), may obtain:

a. (U) "The contents of any wire or electronic communication" held by a provider of remote computing service "on behalf of . . . a subscriber or customer of such remote computing service." 18 U.S.C. § 2703(b)(1)(B)(i), § 2703(b)(2);

b. (U) "The contents of a wire or electronic communication that has been in electronic storage in an electronic communications system for more than one hundred and eighty days." 18 U.S.C. § 2703(a); and

c. (U) Basic subscriber information listed in 18 U.S.C. § 2703(c)(2).

(U)

b2
b7E

(U) **Notice:**

b2
b7E

(U) **Legal standards for delaying notice.** The supervisory official must certify in writing that "there is reason to believe that notification of the existence of the court order may . . . endanger[] the life or physical safety of an individual; [lead to] flight from prosecution; [lead to] destruction of or tampering with evidence; [lead to] intimidation of potential witnesses; or . . . otherwise seriously jeopardiz[e] an investigation or unduly delay[] a trial." 18 U.S.C. §§ 2705(a)(1)(A), 2705(a)(2). Importantly, this standard must be satisfied anew every time an extension of the delayed notice is sought.

8. (U) **Subpoena without Prior Notice to the Subscriber or Customer:** Investigators can subpoena basic subscriber information listed in 18 U.S.C. § 2703(c)(2).

(U) The government may use an administrative subpoena authorized by a federal or state statute or a federal or state grand jury or trial subpoena to compel a provider to disclose basic subscriber information listed in 18 U.S.C. § 2703(c)(2): "name; address; local and long distance telephone connection records, or records of session times and durations; length of service (including start date) and types of service used; telephone or instrument number or other subscriber number or identity, including any temporarily assigned network address; and means and source of payment for such service (including any credit card or bank account number)[.]"

(U)

b2
b7E

See PATRIOT Act § 210, 115 Stat. 272, 283 (2001).

(U) **Legal Standard:** The legal threshold for issuing a subpoena is low. In United States v. Morton Salt Co., 338 U.S. 632, 642-43 (1950), the Court articulated the deferential standard for judicial review of administrative enforcement actions is a four-factor evaluation of "good faith" issuance requiring that: (i) the investigation is conducted pursuant to a legitimate purpose; (ii) the information requested under the subpoena is relevant to that purpose; (iii) the agency does not already have the information it is seeking with the subpoena; and (iv) the agency has followed the necessary administrative steps in issuing the subpoena.

(U//FOUO) In the event that a federal grand jury subpoena is used, however, appropriate protections against disclosure must be followed in compliance with FRCP Rule 6(e).

b2
b7E

Where the telephone billing records being sought are those of a member of the news media, approval of the Attorney General is required. (See DIOG Section 11.9.1.E)

C. (U) Voluntary Disclosure

b2
b7

1. (U) **Service NOT Available to the Public:** Providers of services not available "to the public" are not prohibited from disclosure under ECPA, and so the provider may freely disclose both contents and other records relating to stored communications. Andersen Consulting v. UOP, 991 F. Supp. 1041 (N.D. Ill. 1998) (giving hired consulting firm employees access to UOP's e-mail system is not equivalent to providing e-mail to the public). Only providers of services to the public are prohibited from disclosing stored contents and records, unless statutorily authorized.

2. (U) **Services That ARE Available to the Public:** If the services offered by the provider are available to the public, then ECPA precludes both the disclosure of contents to any third party, including the government, and the disclosure of other records to any governmental entity unless a statutory exception applies. The statutory exceptions permit disclosure by a provider to the public, in essence when the needs of public safety and service providers outweigh privacy interests.

   (U) If the provider is authorized to disclose the information to the government under 18 U.S.C. § 2702 and is willing to do so voluntarily, law enforcement does not need to obtain a legal order to compel the disclosure.

   (U) If a provider voluntarily discloses under the statute, there is no follow-up legal process required or available. If the provider, on the other hand, either may not or will not disclose the information, FBI employees must rely on compelled disclosure provisions and obtain the appropriate legal orders.

   i. (U) **Voluntary disclosure of Stored Contents**

      (U) ECPA authorizes the voluntary disclosure of stored contents when:

      (a) (U) The disclosure is with the consent (express or implied) of the originator, addressee, intended recipient, or the subscriber in the case of opened e-mail, 18 U.S.C. § 2702(b)(3);

      (b) (U) The disclosure "may be necessarily incident to the rendition of the service or to the protection of the rights or property of the provider of that service," 18 U.S.C. § 2702(b)(5);

      (c) (U) The provider "in good faith, believes that an emergency involving danger of death or serious physical injury to any person requires disclosure without delay of information relating to the emergency," 18 U.S.C. § 2702(b)(8);

      (d) (U) To the National Center for Missing and Exploited Children, in connection with a report submitted thereto under Section 227 of the Victims of Child Abuse Act of 1990. (42 U.S.C. § 13032 and 18 U.S.C. § 2702[b][6]); or

      (e) (U) The contents are inadvertently obtained by the service provider and appear to pertain to the commission of a crime. Such disclosures can only be made to a law enforcement agency. 18 U.S.C. § 2702(b)(7)

ii. (U) **Voluntary disclosure of Non-content Customer Records**

(U) ECPA provides for the voluntary disclosure of non-content customer records by a provider to a governmental entity when:

(a) (U) The disclosure is with the consent (express or implied) of the customer or subscriber or 18 U.S.C. § 2702(c)(2) ;

(b) (U) The disclosure "may be necessarily incident to the rendition of the service or to the protection of the rights or property of the provider of that service," 18 U.S.C. § 2702(c)(3);

(c) (U) The provider "in good faith, believes that an emergency involving danger of death or serious physical injury to any person requires disclosure without delay of information relating to the emergency," 18 U.S.C. § 2702(c)(4); or

(U//FOUO) **Note:** an emergency disclosure under this statutory exception is justified when the circumstances demand immediate action on the part of the government to prevent death or serious bodily injury, and does not depend on the immediacy of the risk of danger itself. For example, an e-mail that discusses a planned terrorist attack but not the timing for the attack would constitute an emergency that threatens life or limb, even though the timing of the attack is unknown. It is the need for immediate action to prevent the serious harm threatened by these circumstances rather than the immediacy of the threat itself that is the reason Congress authorized voluntary disclosures under this exception. H.Rpt. No. 107-497 p 13-14 (June 11, 2002) accompanying H.R. 3482, The Cyber Security Enhancement Act of 2002, which passed as part of the comprehensive Homeland Security Act, See P.L. 107-296 § 225.

(d) (U) To the National Center for Missing and Exploited Children, in connection with a report submitted thereto under Section 227 of the Victims of Child Abuse Act of 1990. (42 U.S.C. § 13032 and 18 U.S.C. § 2702[c][5])

iii. (U) **Preservation of Evidence under 18 U.S.C. § 2703(f):**

b2
b7E

(U) A governmental entity is authorized to direct providers to preserve stored records and communications pursuant to 18 U.S.C. § 2703(f).

b2
b7E

Once a preservation request is made, ECPA requires that the provider must retain the records for 90 days, renewable for another 90-day period upon a government request. See 18 U.S.C. § 2703 (f)(2).

(U) Specifically, 18 U.S.C. § 2703(f)(1) states:

(a) (U) A provider of wire or electronic communication service or a remote computing service, upon the request of a governmental entity, must take all necessary steps to preserve records and other evidence in its possession pending the issuance of a court order or other process.

(b) (U) There is no legally prescribed format for 18 U.S.C. § 2703(f) requests.

b2
b7E

(U) FBI employees who send 18 U.S.C. § 2703(f) letters to network service providers should be aware of two limitations. First, the authority to direct providers to preserve records and other evidence is not prospective. That is, 18 U.S.C. § 2703(f) letters can order a provider to preserve records that have already been created but cannot order providers to preserve records not yet made. If FBI employees want providers to record information about future electronic communications, they must comply with the electronic surveillance statutes. A second limitation of 18 U.S.C. § 2703(f) is that some providers may be unable to comply effectively with 18 U.S.C. § 2703(f) requests

b2
b7E

iv. (U) **Video Tape Rental or Sales Records**

(U) Title 18 United States Code Section 2710 makes the unauthorized disclosure of records by any person engaged in the rental, sale, or delivery of prerecorded video cassette tapes or similar audiovisual materials unlawful and provides an exclusionary rule to prohibit personally identifiable information otherwise obtained from being admissible as evidence in any court proceeding. Personally identifiable information is defined as "information that identifies a person as having requested or obtained specific video material or services . . . ."

(a) (U) The disclosure to law enforcement of "personally identifiable information" is permitted only when the law enforcement agency:

(1) (U) Has the written consent of the customer;

(2) (U) Obtains a warrant issued under the FRCP or equivalent state warrant; or

(3) (U) A grand jury subpoena;

(b

b2
b7E

(U) This type of information was specifically not included in the definition of "personally identifiable information" to allow law enforcement to obtain information about individuals during routine investigations such as neighborhood investigations.

(U//FOUO) The disclosure of "personally identifiable information" in a national security case may be compelled through use of the above legal processes or pursuant to a business records order issued under 50 U.S.C. § 1861.

11.10.4. (U) Approval Requirements for Investigative Method

A. (U) Voluntary Emergency Disclosure

(U//FOUO) ECPA protects subscriber and transactional information regarding communications from disclosure by providers of telephone or other electronic communication services. Generally, an NSL, grand jury subpoena, or other form of legal process must be used to compel the communication service provider to disclose such information.

b2
b7E

(U//FOUO)

b2
b7E

(U//FOUO)

b2
b7E

(U//FOUO)

b2
b7E

11.10.5. (U) Duration of Approval

(U) As authorized by statute (e.g., for as long as the emergency necessitating usage exists and only in those circumstances when it is impracticable to obtain legal process) and applicable court order or warrant.

11.10.6. (U//FOUO) Specific Procedures

A. (U//FOUO) Filing requirements:

b2
b7E

b2
b71

B. (U//FOUO) Contact with Providers:

b2
b7E

C. (U) Cost Reimbursement:

(U) Policy and procedures regarding cost reimbursement are described in the following:

(U) Consistent payment procedures

b2
b7E

(U) 5/25/2005 Cost Reimbursement Guidance (18 U.S.C. § 2706 - ECPA)

11.10.7. (U) Notice and Reporting Requirements

A. (U) **Voluntary disclosures:** Title 18 United States Code Section 2702(d) requires the Attorney General to report annually to Congress information pertaining to the receipt of voluntary disclosures of the contents of stored wire or electronic communications in an emergency under 18 U.S.C. § 2702(b)(8), specifically:

1. (U) The number of accounts from which DOJ received voluntary disclosures under subsection (b)(8); and

2. (U) Summary of the basis for disclosure in those instances where the investigation pertaining to those disclosures was closed without the filing of criminal charges.

B. (U) **Roles/Responsibilities:** OGC/ILB is assigned the administrative responsibility to, b December 31 of each year:

1. (U) Tabulate the number of voluntary disclosures of stored contents received under the authority of 18 U.S.C. § 2702(b)(8) for the calendar year;

2. (U) Prepare the report summarizing the basis for disclosure in those instances where the investigation pertaining to those disclosures was closed without the filing of criminal charges; and

3. (U) Submit the report to OGC for review and submission to DOJ according to the statutory requirement for annual report by the Attorney General.

11.10.8. (U) Other Applicable Policies

b2
b7E

11.11. (U) Investigative Method: Pen Registers and Trap and Trace devices in conformity with chapter 206 of Title 18, United States Code, and the Foreign Intelligence Surveillance Act

11.11.1. (U) Summary

(U) Pen register and trap and trace (PR/TT) devices enable the prospective collection of non-content traffic information associated with wire and electronic communications, such as: the phone numbers dialed from or to a particular telephone, including electronic communications; messages sent from or to a particular telephone; or the Internet provider (IP) address of communications on the Internet and other computer networks.

(U//FOUO) **Application:** The PR/TT may be used in preliminary and full national security and criminal investigations. This method may not be used for: (i) targeting a United States person when providing assistance to other agencies, unless there is already an open FBI preliminary or full investigation related to the request for assistance or the predicate exists to open a preliminary or full investigation; (ii) targeting a United States person when collecting against a foreign intelligence requirement; or (iii) during an assessment.

11.11.2. (U) Legal Authority

(U) 18 U.S.C. §§ 3121 et seq. and 50 U.S.C. §§ 1842 et seq. regulate the use of PR/TT devices. PR/TT orders can collect IP addresses, port numbers and the "To" and "From" information from e-mail; they cannot intercept the content of a communication, such as words in the "subject line" or the body of an e-mail.

11.11.3. (U) Definition of Investigative Method

(U) A pen register device records or decodes dialing, routing addressing or signaling information transmitted by an instrument or facility from which a wire or electronic communication is transmitted, provided that such information must not include the contents of any communication. 18 U.S.C. § 3127(3).

(U) A trap and trace device captures the incoming electronic or other impulses that identify the originating number or other dialing, routing, addressing or signaling information reasonably likely to identify the source of a wire or electronic communication, provided that such information does not include the contents of any communication. 18 U.S.C. § 3127(4).

11.11.4. (U) Standards for Use and Approval Requirements for Investigative Method

A. (U) **Pen Register/Trap and Trace under FISA:** Applications for authority to use a PR/TT device can be made to the FISC in national security investigations.

   1. (U) **Legal Standard:** Applications to the FISC are to be under oath and must include:

      a. (U) The identity of the federal officer making the application; and

      b. (U) A certification by the applicant that the information likely to be obtained is foreign intelligence information not concerning a United States person or, if concerning a United States person, is information that is relevant to an ongoing investigation to protect the United States against international terrorism or clandestine intelligence activities; and that such investigation, if of a United States person, is not conducted solely upon the basis of activities protected by the First Amendment to the Constitution.

2. (U//FOUO) **Procedures:** Requests for initiation or renewal of FISA PR/TT must be made using [ ] FISAMS will route the request to appropriate parties for their review and approval of the request [ ] Routing a paper copy for signatures is not required.

b2
b7E

3. (U) **Emergency Authority—FISA:** 50 U.S.C. § 1843

(U//FOUO) Under the provisions of FISA, the Attorney General may grant Emergency Authority (EA) for PR/TT. Requests for Emergency Authority must be referred to the appropriate FBIHQ Division.

(U//FOUO) [ ]

b2
b7E

a. (U) The Attorney General may authorize the installation and use of a PR/TT upon a determination that an emergency exists and that the factual basis exists for a court order. The FISC must be informed at the time of the authorization and an application for a court order must be made to the court no more than seven (7) days after the authorization. Emergency-authorized PR/TT use must terminate when the information sought is obtained, when the FISC denies the application, or seven (7) days after the Attorney General authorization is given.

b. (U) If the FISC denies the application after an emergency PR/TT device has been installed, no information collected as a result may be used in any manner, except with the approval of the Attorney General upon a showing that the information indicates a threat of death or serious bodily harm to any person.

(U) Notwithstanding the foregoing, the President, acting through the Attorney General, may authorize the use of a PR/TT, without a court order, for a period not to exceed 15 calendar days, following a declaration of war by Congress.

(U//FOUO) If an emergency situation arises after regular business hours, [ ] at any time during an emergency.

b2
b7E

B. (U) **Criminal Pen Register/Trap and Trace under 18 U.S.C. §§ 3121 et seq.:** Applications for the installation and use of a PR/TT device may be made to a "court of competent jurisdiction"—i.e., "any district court of the United States (including a magistrate judge of such a court) or any United States court of appeals having jurisdiction over the offense being investigated, or any court of general criminal jurisdiction of a State authorized by the law of that State to enter orders authorizing the use of a pen register or trap and trace device." 18 U.S.C. § 3127(2).

1. (U) **Legal Standard:** Applications for authorization to install and use a PR/TT device must include:

    a. (U) The identity of the attorney for the government or the state law enforcement or investigative officer making the application and the identity of the law enforcement agency conducting the investigation; and

    b. (U) A certification by the applicant that the information likely to be obtained is relevant to an ongoing criminal investigation being conducted by that agency.

2. (U//FOUO) **Procedures:** An SSA must approve a request for initiation or renewal of PR/TT use prior to submission of the request to an attorney for the government. Before approving such a request, the SSA should consider of the following:

    a. (U//FOUO) The use of resources based on the investigative purpose set forth;

    b. (U//FOUO) Whether there is sufficient factual basis for the certification to be made in the application (i.e., is the information likely to be obtained relevant to an ongoing criminal investigation);

    c. (U//FOUO) Whether the customer or subscriber has consented to the use of a PR/TT, see 18 U.S.C. § 3121(b)(3); or

    d. (U//FOUO) Whether the use of a PR/TT is the least intrusive method feasible under the circumstances.

(U//FOUO) A copy of the approving EC must be maintained in the investigative case file and/or sub file and in the ELSUR Administrative Subfile to the corresponding case file.

(U//FOUO) A PR/TT order is executable anywhere within the United States and, upon service, the order applies to any person or entity providing wire or electronic communication service in the United States whose assistance may facilitate the execution of the order. Whenever such an order is served on any person or entity not specifically named in the order, upon request of such person or entity, the attorney for the government or law enforcement or investigative officer that is serving the order must provide written or electronic certification that the order applies to the person or entity being served.

3. (U) **Emergency Authority—Criminal:**

(U) The Attorney General, the Deputy Attorney General, the Associate Attorney General, any Assistant Attorney General, any acting Assistant Attorney General, or any Deputy Assistant Attorney General may specially designate any investigative or law enforcement officer to determine whether an emergency situation that requires the installation and use of a PR/TT device before an order authorizing such installation and use can, with due diligence, be obtained.

(U) An emergency situation as defined in this section involves:

a. (U) Immediate danger of death or serious bodily injury to any person;

b. (U) Conspiratorial activities characteristic of organized crime;

c. (U) An immediate threat to a national security interest; or

d. (U) An ongoing attack on a protected computer (as defined in 18 U.S.C. § 1030) that constitutes a crime punishable by a term of imprisonment greater than one year.

(U) If the DOJ authorizes the emergency installation of a PR/TT, the government has 48 hours after the installation to apply for a court order according to 18 U.S.C. § 3123. It is a violation of law to fail to apply for a court order within this 48 hour period. Use of the PR/TT shall immediately terminate when the information sought is obtained, when the application for a court order is denied, or if no court order has been obtained 48 hours after the installation of the PR/TT device.

(U//FOUO) As with requesting authorization for an emergency Title III,

b2
b7E

Once that approval has been obtained, the DOJ attorney will advise the AUSA that the emergency use has been approved and that the law enforcement agency may proceed with the installation and use of the PR/TT. The DOJ attorney will send a verification memorandum, signed by the authorizing official, to the AUSA. The AUSA will include an authorization memorandum with the application for the court order approving the emergency use.

(U//FOUO) If an emergency situation arises after regular business hours,

During regular business hours,

b2
b7E

11.11.5. (U) Duration of Approval

(U) **National Security:** The use of a PR/TT device may be authorized by the FISC for a period of time not to exceed 90 days in cases targeting a United States person. Extensions may be granted for periods not to exceed 90 days upon re-application to the court. In cases targeting a non-United States person, an order or extension may be for a period of time not to exceed one year.

(U) **Criminal:** The installation and use of a PR/TT device may be authorized by court order under 18 U.S.C. § 3123 for a period not to exceed sixty days, which may be extended for additional sixty-day periods.

11.11.6. (U//FOUO) Specific Procedures

A. (U//FOUO) Prior to installing and using a PR/TT device (whether issued in a criminal or national security matter), the case agent should:

1. (U//FOUO

b2
b7E

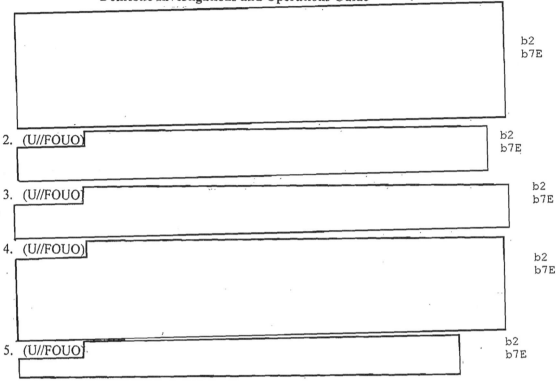

b2
b7E

2. (U//FOUO)   b2
b7E

3. (U//FOUO)   b2
b7E

4. (U//FOUO)   b2
b7E

5. (U//FOUO)   b2
b7E

11.11.7. (U) Use and Dissemination of Information Derived from Pen Register/Trap and Trace Authorized Pursuant to FISA

(U) 50 U.S.C. § 1845

A. (U) No information acquired from a PR/TT device installed and used pursuant to FISA may be used or disclosed by federal officers or employees except for lawful purposes.

B. (U) No information acquired pursuant to a FISA authorized PR/TT may be disclosed for law enforcement purposes unless such disclosure is accompanied by a statement that such information, or any information derived therefrom, may only be used in a criminal proceeding with the advance authorization of the Attorney General.

C. (U) Whenever the United States intends to enter into evidence or otherwise use or disclose in any trial, hearing, or other proceeding in or before any court, department, officer, agency, regulatory body, or other authority of the United States against an aggrieved person any information obtained or derived from the use of a PR/TT device acquired pursuant to FISA, the United States must, before the trial, hearing, or other proceeding or at a reasonable time before an effort to so disclose or so use that information or submit it into evidence, notify the aggrieved person, and the court or other authority in which the information is to be disclosed or used, that the United States intends to so disclose or so use such information.

(U) Note: 50 U.S.C. § 1801(k) defines aggrieved person as: "a person who is the target of an electronic surveillance or any other person whose communications or activities were subject to electronic surveillance."

11.11.8. (U) Notice and Reporting Requirements

A. (U) **Annual Report for Criminal Pen Register/Trap and Trace**: The Attorney General is required to make an annual report to Congress on the number of criminal PR/TT orders applied for by DOJ law enforcement agencies. 18 U.S.C. § 3126. The report is to include the following information:

1. (U) The period of interceptions authorized by the order, and the number and duration of any extensions;

2. (U) The offense specified in the order or application, or extension;

3. (U) The number of investigations involved;

4. (U) The number and nature of the facilities affected; and

5. (U) The identity, including the district, of the applying agency making the application and the person authorizing the order.

(U//FOUO) DOJ, Criminal Division, Office of Enforcement Operations requires that the FBI provide quarterly reports on pen register usage. To satisfy DOJ data requirements and standardize and simplify field reporting, Court-ordered pen register usage must be reported to FBIHQ[   ]within five workdays of the expiration date of an original order or extensions, or denial of an application for an order. For all criminal PR/TT orders or extensions issued on or after January 1, 2009[   ][   ]These reporting requirements do not apply to PR/TT authorized pursuant to consent or under the provisions of FISA.

b2
b7E

B. (U) **Semi-Annual Report for National Security Pen Registers and Trap and Trace**: The Attorney General must inform the House Permanent Select Committee on Intelligence, Senate Select Committee on Intelligence, Committee of the Judiciary of the House Representatives, and Committee of the Judiciary of the Senate concerning all uses of PR/TT devices pursuant to 50 U.S.C. § 1846. This report is coordinated through DOJ NSD. A semi-annual report must be submitted that contains the following information:

1. (U) The total number of applications made for orders approving the use of PR/TT devices;

2. (U) The total number of such orders either granted, modified, or denied; and

3. (U) The total number of PR/TT devices whose installation and use was authorized by the Attorney General on an emergency basis and the total number of subsequent orders approving or denying the installation and use of such PR/TT devices.

11.11.9. (U) Special Circumstances

A. (U//FOUO) **Avoiding Collection and Investigative Use of "Content" in the Operation of Pen Registers and Trap and Trace Devices**

1. (U//FOUO) **Overview**: Telecommunication networks provide users the ability to engage in extended dialing and/or signaling, (also known as "post cut-through dialed digits" or PCTDD), which in some circumstances are simply call-routing information and, in others, are call content. For example, PCTDD occur when a party places a calling card, credit card, or collect call by first dialing a long-distance carrier access number and then, after the initial call is "cut through," dials the telephone number of the destination party. In

other instances, PCTDD may represent call content, such as when a party calls an automated banking service and enters an account number, calls a pharmacy's automated prescription refill service and enters prescription information, or enters a call-back number when prompted by a voice mail service. See United States Telecom Assn v. Federal Communications Commission, 227 F.3d 450, 462 (D.C. Cir. 2000)

b2
b7E

(U//FOUO) The definition of both a pen register device and a trap and trace device provides that the information collected by these devices "shall not include the contents of any communication." 18 U.S.C. § 3127. In addition, 18 U.S.C. § 3121(c) makes explicit the requirement to "use technology reasonably available" that restricts the collection of information "so as not to include the contents of any wire or electronic communications." "Content" includes any information concerning the substance, purpose, or meaning of a communication. 18 U.S.C. § 2510(8). When the pen register definition is read in conjunction with the limitation provision, however, it suggests that although a PR/TT device may not be used for the express purpose of collecting content, the incidental collection of content may occur despite the use of "reasonably available" technology to minimize, to the extent feasible, any possible over collection of content while still allowing the device to collect all of the dialing and signaling information authorized.

DOJ Policy: In addition to this statutory obligation, DOJ has issued a directive to all DOJ agencies requiring that no affirmative investigative use may be made of PCTDD incidentally collected that constitutes content, except in cases of emergency—to prevent an immediate danger of death, serious physical injury, or harm to the national security.

(U//FOUO)

b2
b7E

2. (U//FOUO) Collection:

b2
b7E

a. (U//FOUO)

b2
b7E

b2
b7E

b. (U//FOUO)

b2
b7E

3. (U//FOUO) **Use of PCTDD:**

b2
b7E

a. (U//FOUO)

b2
b7E

i. (U//FOUO)

b2
b7E

ii. (U//FOUO)

b2
b7E

(U//FOUO)

b2
b7E

iii. (U//FOUO)

b2
b7E

iv. (U//FOUO)

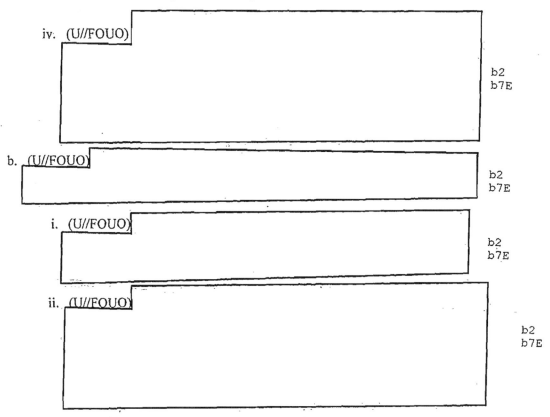

b2
b7E

b. (U//FOUO)

b2
b7E

i. (U//FOUO)

b2
b7E

ii. (U//FOUO)

b2
b7E

4. (U//FOUO) **What constitutes PCTDD content:** In applying the above, the term "content" is interpreted to mean "any information concerning the substance, purpose, or meaning of a communication" as defined in 18 U.S.C. § 2510. Questions concerning whether specific PCTDD are content as opposed to dialing, routing or signaling information should be addressed to the CDC or OGC for coordination with DOJ as necessary.

(U//FOUO)

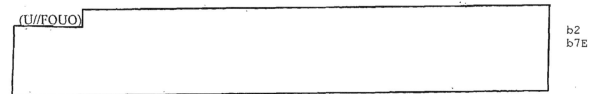

b2
b7E

B. (U//FOUO) **Use of cell site simulators/digital analyzers/wireless intercept tracking technology.** A PR/TT order or consent is required for the FBI to use equipment to capture any "signaling information"—including the Mobile Station Identification Number (MSIN) and Electronic Serial Number (ESN) or other registration-type data—emitted from a wireless phone into the public airspace—even though this can be accomplished without the assistance of the service provider. Because 18 U.S.C. § 3127 defines PR/TT devices in terms of recording, decoding or capturing dialing, routing, addressing, or signaling information, the government's use of its own device to capture such signaling data—whether passively monitoring or actively interrogating—constitutes the use of a "pen register" device and requires an order or statutory exception to avoid violating the statute. The following discusses how wireless intercept tracking technology (WITT) is used:

1. (U//FOUO) **To Locate a Known Phone:**

   a. (U//FOUO) **Authority:** A standard PR/TT order is adequate to authorize the use of this technology to determine the location of a known targeted phone, provided that the language authorizes FBI employees to install or cause to be installed and use a pen register device, without geographical limitation, at any time of day or night within (X) days from the date the order is signed, to record or decode dialing, routing, addressing, or signaling information transmitted by the "Subject Telephone." The application and order should generally also request authority to compel disclosure of cell site location data on an ongoing basis under 18 U.S.C. § 2703(d)—or probable cause, if such is required by the particular district court—as such information may assist in determining the general location of the targeted phone.

   b. (U//FOUO)

   c. (U//FOUO)

   Under <u>Kyllo v. United States,</u> 533 U.S. 27 (2001), the use of equipment not in general public use to acquire data that is not otherwise detectable that emanates from a private premise implicates the Fourth Amendment.

   (U//FOUO)

b2
b7E

2. (U//FOUO) **To Identify an Unknown Target Phone Number:**

(U//FOUO) Authority:

b2
b7E

(U//FOUO)

b2
b7E

a. (U//FOUO)

b2
b7E

b. (U//FOUO)

b2
b7E

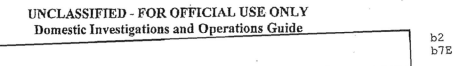

b2
b7E

C. (U) **PR/TT Order Language:** The language in the order should state that "the pen register will be implemented unobtrusively and with minimum interference with the services accorded to customers of such service."

11.12. (U) Investigative Method: Electronic Surveillance under Title III and under FISA

11.12.1. (U) Summary

(U//FOUO) Electronic Surveillance (ELSUR) is a valuable investigative method. It is, also, a very intrusive means of acquiring information relevant to the effective execution of the FBI's law enforcement, national security and intelligence missions. To ensure that due consideration is given to the competing interests between law enforcement and the effect on privacy and civil liberties, this section contains various administrative and management controls beyond those imposed by statute and DOJ guidelines. Unless otherwise noted, it is the responsibility of the case agent and his/her supervisor to ensure compliance with these instructions. ELSUR is only authorized as an investigative method in the conduct of full investigations. ELSUR requires: (i) administrative or judicial authorization prior to its use; (ii) contact with the Field Office ELSUR Technician to coordinate all necessary recordkeeping; and (iii) consultation with the Technical Advisor (TA) or a designated TTA to determine feasibility, applicability, and use of the appropriate equipment.

(U//FOUO) **Application:**

b2
b7E

11.12.2. (U) Legal Authority

(U) ELSUR is authorized by chapter 119, 18 U.S.C. §§ 2510-2522 (Title III of the Omnibus and Safe Streets Act of 1968); 50 U.S.C. §§ 1801-1811 (FISA); and E.O. 12333 § 2.5.

11.12.3. (U) Definition of Investigative Method

(U) ELSUR is the non-consensual electronic collection of information (usually communications) under circumstances in which the parties have a reasonable expectation of privacy and court orders or warrants are required.

11.12.4. (U) Standards for Use and Approval Requirements for Investigative Method

A. (U//FOUO) **FISA**

1. (U//FOUO) FBIHQ and Field Office requests for FISC ELSUR orders must use the FISA Request Form. Field Office requests for FISA orders are submitted and tracked through FISAMS. The FISA request forms, in a question and answer format, have been designed to ensure that all information needed for the preparation of a FISC application is provided to FBIHQ and to the DOJ.

2. (U) A Certification by the Director of the FBI or one of nine other individuals authorized by Congress or the President to provide such certifications that the information being sought is foreign intelligence information; that a significant purpose of the electronic surveillance is to obtain foreign intelligence information; that such

information cannot reasonably be obtained by normal investigative techniques; that the information sought is "foreign intelligence information" as defined by FISA; and includes a statement explaining the certifier's basis for the certification.

(U) **Note:** Title 50 of the United States Code Section 1804 specifies the Assistant to the President for National Security Affairs; E.O. 12139 as amended by E.O. 13383 specifies the Director of the FBI, Deputy Director of the FBI, the Director of National Intelligence, the Principal Deputy Director of National Intelligence, the Director of the Central Intelligence Agency, the Secretary of State, the Deputy Secretary of State, the Secretary of Defense, and the Deputy Secretary of Defense as appropriate officials to make certifications required by FISA.

3. (U) Emergency FISA Authority (50 U.S.C. § 1805[f])

(U) The Attorney General, on request from the Director of the FBI or his/her designee, may authorize an emergency FISA for electronic surveillance when it is reasonably determined that an emergency situation exists that precludes advance FISC review and approval and that a factual predication for the issuance of a FISA Order exists. A FISC judge must be informed by DOJ at the time of the emergency authorization and an application must be submitted to that judge as soon as is practicable but not more than seven (7) days after the emergency authority has been approved by the Attorney General. If a court order is denied after an emergency surveillance has been initiated, no information gathered as a result of the surveillance may be used as evidence or disclosed in any trial or other proceeding, and no information concerning any United States person acquired from such surveillance may be used or disclosed in any manner, except with the approval of the Attorney General if the information indicates a threat of death or serious bodily harm to any person.

(U//FOUO) For an emergency FISA for electronic surveillance

at any time.

b2
b7E

B. (U) **Title III**

(U//FOUO) An SAC (or designee) has the authority to approve requests for "non-sensitive" Title III orders. An Acting SAC may approve such requests in the absence of the SAC. The authority to approve Title III applications may not be delegated lower than the ASAC level. The SAC, with the recommendation of the CDC, must determine whether the request involves sensitive circumstances.

(U//FOUO) If a Title III involves one of the seven "sensitive circumstances," it must be approved by FBIHQ.

(U//FOUO) The following five sensitive circumstances require the approval of a Deputy Assistant Director (DAD) or higher from the Criminal Investigative Division (CID), Counterintelligence Division (CD), or Counterterrorism Division (CTD), as appropriate:

1. (U//FOUO) Significant privilege issues or First Amendment concerns (e.g., attorney-client privilege or other privileged conversations or interception of news media representatives);

2. (U//FOUO) Significant privacy concerns (e.g., interceptions of conversations in a bedroom or bathroom);

3. (U//FOUO) Applications based on "relaxed specificity" (i.e., "roving" interception) under 18 U.S.C. § 2518(11)(a) and (b);

4. (U//FOUO) Applications concerning Domestic Terrorism, International Terrorism, or Espionage investigations; or

5. (U//FOUO) Any situation deemed appropriate by the AD of CID or OGC.

(U//FOUO) The following two sensitive circumstances require the approval of the Director, the Acting Director, Deputy Director, or the EAD for the Criminal Cyber Response and Services Branch, or the EAD for the National Security Branch, or the respective Assistant Director for Counterterrorism or Counterintelligence:

6. (U//FOUO) "Emergency" Title III interceptions (i.e., interceptions conducted prior to judicial approval under 18 U.S.C. § 2518[7]); or

7. (U//FOUO) The interception of communications of members of Congress, federal judges, high-level federal officials, high-level state executives, or members of a state judiciary or legislature is anticipated.

(U//FOUO) All requests for electronic surveillance that involve one of the above "sensitive circumstances" must be reviewed by the OGC prior to approval.

(U//FOUO) With the prior approval of the Attorney General, or Attorney General's designee, the United States Attorney or the Strike Force Attorney must apply to a federal judge for a court order authorizing the interception of communications relating to one or more of the offenses listed in Title III (18 U.S.C. § 2516). Judicial oversight continues into the operational phase of the electronic surveillance—installation, monitoring, transcribing and handling of recording media.

(U//FOUO) An extension order may be sought to continue monitoring beyond the initial 30-day period without a lapse in time. When a break in coverage has occurred, a renewal order may be sought to continue monitoring the same interceptees or facilities identified in the original authorization. The affidavit and application in support of an extension or renewal must comply with all of the Title III requirements, including approval of the Attorney General or designee. Except as explained below, extensions that occur within 30 days of the original Title III order do not require review by the SAC or designee. After a lapse of more than 30 days, the SAC or designee must review and request renewed electronic surveillance.

(U//FOUO) There may be situations or unusual circumstances that require the FBI to adopt an already existing Title III from another federal law enforcement agency. This will be approved on a case-by-case basis, only in exceptional circumstances.

(U//FOUO) Before the FBI begins or adopts the administration of a Title III, the Field Office must obtain SAC or designee approval. Thereafter, extensions and renewals within 30 days do not require SAC or designee approval.

(U//FOUO) Emergency Title III interceptions (e.g., interceptions conducted prior to judicial approval under 18 U.S.C. § 2518[7]) – [Hyperlink to Memo dated May 22. 2008 Standard and Process Authorization]

(U//FOUO) If an emergency situation arises after regular business hours [   ]　　　b2
　　b7E

[During regular business hours   ] may be reached

(U//FOUO) **Dispute Resolution for both FISA and Title III Applications**

(U//FOUO) [   ]　　　b2
　　b7E

11.12.5.　(U) Duration of Approval

A. (U) FISA

(U//FOUO) FISC orders for ELSUR surveillance are provided for the period of time specified in the order that will not exceed: 90 days for United States persons; 120 days for non-United States persons; and one year for a foreign power, as defined in 50 U.S.C. § 1801(a) (1)(2) or (3). For United States persons, renewals of FISA Orders may be requested for the same period of time originally authorized based upon a continued showing of probable cause. For non-United States persons, renewals can be for a period not to exceed one year. All renewal requests should be submitted to DOJ NSD by the requesting Field Office at least 45 days prior to the expiration of the existing order. These requests are to be submitted using the FISA Request Form process in FISAMS.

B. (U) Title III

(U) Title III ELSUR orders are for a period not to exceed 30 days, with subsequent 30 day extensions as authorized by the court.

11.12.6.　(U) Specific Procedures

A. (U) FISA

b2
b7E

(U//FOUO) [   ]

1.　(U//FOUO) **FISA Verification of Accuracy Procedures**

(U//FOUO) [   ]　　　b2
　　　　　　　　　　　　　　　　　　　　　　　　　　　　　　　　　　　　　b7E

a.　(U//FOUO) [   ]　　　b2
　　　　　　　　　　　　　　　　　　　　　　　　　　　　　　　　　　　b7E

i.　(U//FOUO) [   ]　　　b2
　　　　　　　　　　　　　　　　　　　　　　　　　　　　　　　　　b7E

ii. (U//FOUO) [redacted]   b2
                            b7E

iii. (U//FOUO) [redacted]   b2
                            b7E

b. (U//FOUO) [redacted]   b2
                            b7E

2. (U//FOUO) **FISA Electronic Surveillance Administrative Sub-file**

(U//FOUO) [redacted]   b2
                            b7E

a. (U//FOUO) [redacted]   b2
                            b7E

b. (U//FOUO) [redacted]   b2
                            b7E

3. (U//FOUO) **FISA Review Board for FISA Renewals**

(U//FOUO) [redacted]   b2
                            b7E

a. (U//FOUO) [redacted]   b2
                            b7E

b. (U//FOUO) [redacted]   b2
                            b7E

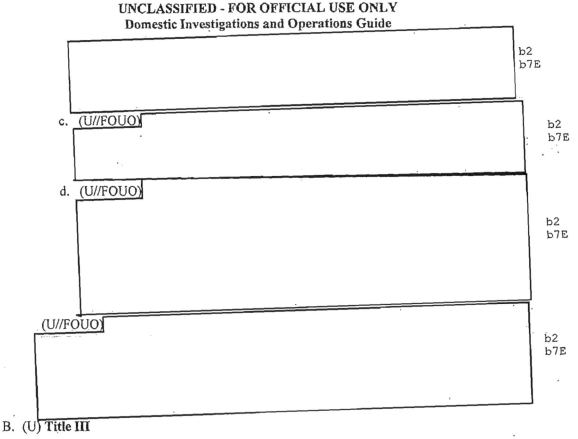

b2
b7E

c. (U//FOUO)

b2
b7E

d. (U//FOUO)

b2
b7E

(U//FOUO)

b2
b7E

B. (U) Title III

1. (U//FOUO) The requirements in 18 U.S.C. § 2518 must be followed meticulously in the preparation of a Title III application. In addition, the following points must be covered:

 a. (U//FOUO) Probable cause must be current;

 b. (U//FOUO) There must be a factual basis for concluding that normal investigative procedures have been tried and failed or a demonstration why these procedures appear to be unlikely to succeed or would be too dangerous if tried ("boilerplate" statements in this respect are unacceptable);

 c. (U//FOUO) If the subscriber of the telephone on which coverage is sought is not one of the principals, attempts to identify the subscriber must be made;

 d. (U//FOUO) Minimization will be occur, as statutorily required, if the coverage involves a public telephone booth, a restaurant table, or the like;

 e. (U//FOUO) The facility or premises to be covered is described fully,   and

b2
b7E

 f. (U//FOUO) At least 10 days prior to submitting the Title III request to DOJ OEO, the Field Office must forward an electronic communication to FBIHQ

b2
b7E

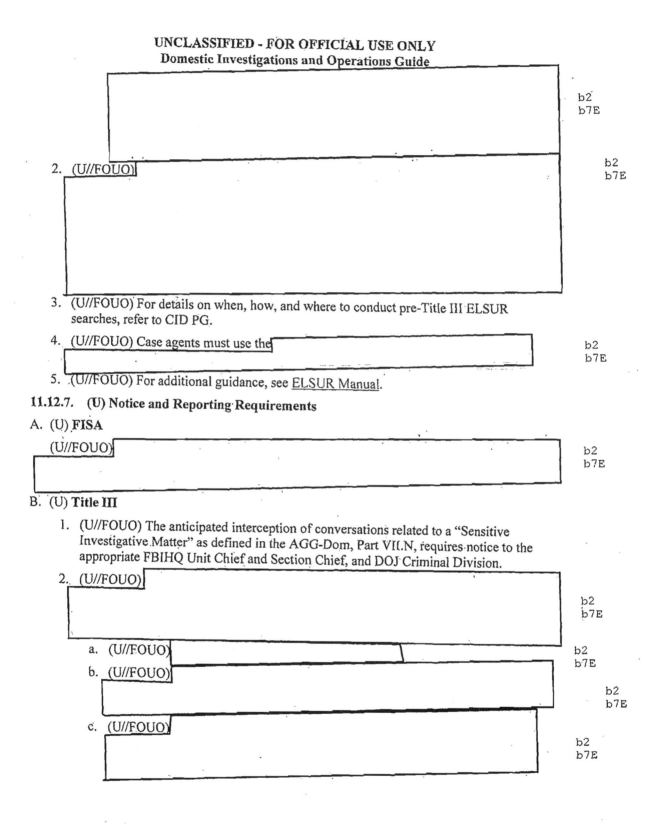

2. (U//FOUO)

b2
b7E

b2
b7E

3. (U//FOUO) For details on when, how, and where to conduct pre-Title III ELSUR searches, refer to CID PG.

4. (U//FOUO) Case agents must use the

b2
b7E

5. (U//FOUO) For additional guidance, see ELSUR Manual.

11.12.7. (U) Notice and Reporting Requirements

A. (U) FISA

(U//FOUO)

b2
b7E

B. (U) Title III

1. (U//FOUO) The anticipated interception of conversations related to a "Sensitive Investigative Matter" as defined in the AGG-Dom, Part VII.N, requires notice to the appropriate FBIHQ Unit Chief and Section Chief, and DOJ Criminal Division.

2. (U//FOUO)

b2
b7E

   a. (U//FOUO)

b2
b7E

   b. (U//FOUO)

b2
b7E

   c. (U//FOUO)

b2
b7E

3. (U//FOUO) [redacted]   b2
                                                               b7E

4. (U//FOUO) [redacted]   b2
                                                               b7E

5. (U//FOUO) Upon completion of a Title III ELSUR activity, the Form 2 report is required to be submitted per 18 U.S.C. § 2519. For details on the completion and submission of the Form 2 report, see the CID PG.

11.12.8. (U) Compliance and Monitoring

A. (U) FISA   b2
                                                               b7E

   (U//FOUO) [redacted]

B. (U) Title III

   (U//FOUO) Upon completion of Title III ELSUR activity, the Form 2 report is required to be submitted per 18 U.S.C. § 2519. For details on the completion and submission of the Form 2 report, see the CID PG.

11.12.9. (U) Special Circumstances

(U) FISA

(U) Under 50 U.S.C. § 1802, the President, through the Attorney General, may authorize electronic surveillance under FISA without a court order for periods of up to one year, if the Attorney General certifies in writing under oath that the surveillance will be solely directed at acquiring communications that are transmitted by means that are exclusively between or among foreign powers and there is no substantial likelihood of the surveillance acquiring the contents of communications to which United States Persons are parties.

11.12.10. (U) Other Applicable Policies

A. (U) FISA

   1. (U//FOUO) CD Policy Guide

   2. (U//FOUO) CTD Policy Guide

   3. (U//FOUO) Investigative Law Unit Library

   4. (U//FOUO) Foreign Intelligence Surveillance Act (FISA) Unit

B. (U//FOUO) OTD PG

   1. (U//FOUO) Title III

   2. (U//FOUO) Memo dated May 22, 2008 Standard and Process Authorization

   3. (U//FOUO) ELSUR Manual

   4. (U//FOUO) CID PG

   5. (U//FOUO) OTD PG

11.13. (U) Investigative Method: Physical searches, including mail openings, requiring judicial order or warrant

(U) AGG-Dom, Part V.A.12.

11.13.1. (U) Summary

(U) The Fourth Amendment to the United States Constitution governs all searches and seizures by government agents. The Fourth Amendment contains two clauses. The first establishes the prohibition against unreasonable searches and seizures. The second provides that no warrant (authorizing a search or seizure) will be issued unless based on probable cause. An unlawful search does not preclude a prosecution. The remedy to the defendant for an unlawful search is suppression of the evidence resulting from the illegal seizure.

(U//FOUO) Application:

b2
b7E

(U) A search is a government invasion of a person's privacy. To qualify as reasonable expectation of privacy, the individual must have an actual subjective expectation of privacy and society must be prepared to recognize that expectation as objectively reasonable. See Katz v. United States, 389 U.S. at 361. The ability to conduct a physical search in an area or situation where an individual has a reasonable expectation of privacy requires a warrant or order issued by a court of competent jurisdiction or an exception to the requirement for such a warrant or order. The warrant or order must be based on probable cause. The United States Supreme Court defines probable cause to search as a "fair probability that contraband or evidence of a crime will be found in a particular place." Illinois v. Gates, 462 U.S. 213, 238 (1983). A government agent may conduct a search without a warrant based on an individual's voluntary consent. A search based on exigent circumstances may also be conducted without a warrant, but the requirement for probable cause remains.

11.13.2. (U) Legal Authority

(U) Searches conducted by the FBI must be in conformity with FRCP Rule 41; FISA, 50 U.S.C. §§ 1821-1829; or E.O. 12333 § 2.5.

11.13.3. (U) Definition of Investigative Method

(U) A physical search constitutes any physical intrusion within the United States into premises or property (including examination of the interior of property by technical means) that is intended to result in the seizure, reproduction, inspection, or alteration of information, material, or property, under circumstances in which a person has a reasonable expectation of privacy.

(U) A physical search requiring a warrant does not include: (i) electronic surveillance as defined in FISA or Title III; or (ii) the acquisition by the United States Government of foreign intelligence information from international foreign communications, or foreign intelligence activities conducted according to otherwise applicable federal law involving a foreign electronic communications system, using a means other than electronic surveillance as defined in FISA.

A. (U) **Requirement for Reasonableness.** By the terms of the Fourth Amendment, a search must be reasonable at its inception and reasonable in its execution.

B. (U) **Reasonable Expectation of Privacy.** The right of privacy is a personal right, not a property concept. It safeguards whatever an individual reasonably expects to be private. The protection normally includes persons, residences, vehicles, other personal property, private conversations, private papers and records. The Supreme Court has determined that there is no reasonable expectation of privacy in certain areas or information. As a result, government intrusions into those areas do not constitute a search and, thus, do not have to meet the requirements of the Fourth Amendment. These areas include: (i) open fields; (ii) prison cells; (iii) public access areas; and (iv) vehicle identification numbers. The Supreme Court has also determined that certain governmental practices do not involve an intrusion into a reasonable expectation of privacy and, therefore, do not amount to a search. These practices include: (i) aerial surveillance conducted from navigable airspace; (ii) field test of suspected controlled substance; and (iii) odor detection. A reasonable expectation of privacy may be terminated by an individual taking steps to voluntarily relinquish the expectation of privacy, such as abandoning property or setting trash at the edge of the curtilage or beyond for collection.

C. (U) **Issuance of search warrant**

1. (U) Under FRCP Rule 41, upon the request of a federal law enforcement officer or an attorney for the government, a search warrant may be issued by:

    a. (U) a federal magistrate judge, or if none is reasonably available, a judge of a state court of record within the federal district, for a search of property or for a person within the district;

    b. (U) a federal magistrate judge for a search of property or for a person either within or outside the district if the property or person is within the district when the warrant is sought but might move outside the district before the warrant is executed;

    c. (U) a federal magistrate judge in any district in which activities related to the terrorism may have occurred, for a search of property or for a person within or outside the district, in an investigation of domestic terrorism or international terrorism (as defined in 18 U.S.C. § 2331); and

    d. (U) a magistrate with authority in the district to issue a warrant to install a tracking device. The warrant may authorize use of the device to track the movement of a person or property located within the district, outside, or both.

2. (U) Physical searches related to a national security purpose may be authorized by the FISC. (50 U.S.C. §§ 1821-1829)

D. (U) Property or Persons That May be Seized with a Warrant.

(U) A warrant may be issued to search for and seize any: (i) property that constitutes evidence of the commission of a criminal offense; (ii) contraband, the fruits of crime, or things otherwise criminally possessed; or (iii) property designed or intended for use or that is or has been used as the means of committing a criminal offense. In addition to a conventional search conducted following issuance of a warrant, examples of search warrants include:

1. **(U) Anticipatory Warrants**

   (U) As the name suggests, an anticipatory warrant differs from other search warrants in that it is not supported by probable cause to believe that contraband exists at the premises to be searched at the time the warrant is issued. Instead, an anticipatory search warrant is validly issued where there is probable cause to believe that a crime has been or is being committed, and that evidence of such crime will be found at the described location at the time of the search, but only after certain specified events transpire. These conditions precedent to the execution of an anticipatory warrant, sometimes referred to as "triggering events," are integral to its validity. Because probable cause for an anticipatory warrant is contingent on the occurrence of certain expected or "triggering" events, typically the future delivery, sale, or purchase of contraband, the judge making the probable cause determination must take into account the likelihood that the triggering event will occur on schedule and as predicted. Should these triggering events fail to materialize, the anticipatory warrant is void.

2. **(U) Sneak and peek search warrants**

   (U) A sneak and peek search warrant allows law enforcement agents to surreptitiously enter a location such as a building, an apartment, garage, storage shed, etc., for the purpose of looking for and documenting evidence of criminal activity. The purpose of this type of warrant is to search for and seize property (either tangible or intangible) without immediately providing notice of the search and a return on the warrant to the owner of the property searched or seized. See FRCP 41(f)(3). A sneak and peek warrant is used to gather additional evidence of criminal activity without prematurely exposing an on-going investigation. The evidence discovered during a sneak and peek search may be used to support a request for a conventional search warrant.

3. **(U) Mail Openings**

   (U) Mail in United States postal channels may be searched only pursuant to court order, or presidential authorization. United States Postal Service regulations governing such activities must be followed. A search of items that are being handled by individual couriers, or commercial courier companies, under circumstances in which there is a reasonable expectation of privacy, or have been sealed for deposit into postal channels, and that are discovered within properties or premises being searched, must be carried out according to unconsented FISA or FRCP Rule 41 physical search procedures.

4. **(U) Compelled Disclosure of the Contents of Stored Wire or Electronic Communications**

   (U) Contents in "electronic storage" (e.g., unopened e-mail/voice mail) require a search warrant. See 18 U.S.C. § 2703(a). A distinction is made between the contents of communications that are in electronic storage (e.g., unopened e-mail) for less than 180 days and those in "electronic storage" for longer than 180 days, or those that are no longer in "electronic storage" (e.g., opened e-mail). In enacting the ECPA, Congress concluded that customers may not retain a "reasonable expectation of privacy" in information sent to network providers. However, the contents of an e-mail message that is unopened should nonetheless be protected by Fourth Amendment standards, similar to the contents of a regularly mailed letter. On the other hand, if the contents of an unopened message are kept beyond six months or stored on behalf of the customer after the e-mail has been received or opened, it should be treated the same as a business record in the hands of a third party, such as an accountant or attorney. In that case, the government may subpoena the records from the third party without running afoul of either the Fourth or Fifth Amendment. If a search warrant is used, it may be served on the provider without notice to the customer or subscriber.

11.13.4. (U) Approval Requirements for Investigative Method

A. (U//FOUO) **Search warrants issued under authority of FRCP Rule 41:** A warrant to search is issued by a federal magistrate (or a state court judge if a federal magistrate is not reasonably available). Coordination with the USAO or DOJ is required to obtain the warrant.

B. (U//FOUO) **FISA:** In national security investigations, Field Office requests for FISA authorized physical searches must be submitted to FBIHQ using the FBI FISA Request Form. Field Office requests for FISA approval are tracked through FISAMS. This form should be completed by the case agent.

C. (U//FOUO) **Sensitive Investigative Matter:** Notice to the appropriate FBIHQ substantive Unit Chief and Section Chief is required if the matter under investigation is a sensitive investigative matter. Notice to DOJ is also required, as described in DIOG Section 10.

11.13.5. (U) Duration of Approval

(U) The duration for the execution of a warrant is established by the court order or warrant.

11.13.6. (U) Specific Procedures

A. (U) **Obtaining a Warrant under FRCP Rule 41**

(U) **Probable Cause.** After receiving an affidavit or other information, a magistrate judge or a judge of a state court of record must issue the warrant if there is probable cause to search for and seize a person or property under FRCP Rule 41(c). Probable cause exists where "the facts and circumstances within the FBI employee's knowledge, and of which they had reasonably trustworthy information are sufficient in themselves to warrant a person of reasonable caution in the belief that..." a crime has been or is being committed, and that seizable property can be found at the place or on the person to be searched. Probable cause is a reasonable belief grounded on facts. In judging whether a reasonable belief exists, the test is whether such a belief would be engendered in a prudent person with the officer's training and experience. To establish probable cause, the affiant must demonstrate a basis for knowledge and belief that the facts are true and that there is probable cause to believe the items listed in the affidavit will be found at the place to be searched.

1. (U) **Requesting a Warrant in the Presence of a Judge.**

    a. (U) **Warrant on an Affidavit:** When a federal law enforcement officer or an attorney for the government presents an affidavit in support of a warrant, the judge may require the affiant to appear personally and may examine under oath the affiant and any witness the affiant produces.

b. (U) **Warrant on Sworn Testimony:** The judge may wholly or partially dispense with a written affidavit and base a warrant on sworn testimony if doing so is reasonable under the circumstances.

c. (U) **Recording Testimony:** Testimony taken in support of a warrant must be recorded by a court reporter or by a suitable recording device, and the judge must file the transcript or recording with the clerk, along with any affidavit.

2. (U) **Requesting a Warrant by Telephonic or Other Means**

a. (U) **In General:** A magistrate judge may issue a warrant based on information communicated by telephone or other appropriate means, including facsimile transmission.

b. (U) **Recording Testimony:** Upon learning that an applicant is requesting a warrant, a magistrate judge must: (i) place under oath the applicant and any person on whose testimony the application is based; and (ii) make a verbatim record of the conversation with a suitable recording device, if available, or by a court reporter, or in writing.

c. (U) **Certifying Testimony:** The magistrate judge must have any recording or court reporter's notes transcribed, certify the transcription's accuracy, and file a copy of the record and the transcription with the clerk. Any written verbatim record must be signed by the magistrate judge and filed with the clerk.

d. (U) **Suppression Limited**: Absent a finding of bad faith, evidence obtained from a warrant issued under FRCP Rule 41(d)(3)(A) is not subject to suppression on the ground that issuing the warrant in that manner was unreasonable under the circumstances.

3. (U) **Issuing the Warrant**

(U) In general, the magistrate judge or a judge of a state court of record must issue the warrant to an officer authorized to execute it. The warrant must identify the person or property to be searched, identify any person or property to be seized, and designate the magistrate judge to whom it must be returned. The warrant must command the officer to: (i) execute the warrant within a specified time no longer than 10 days; (ii) execute the warrant during the daytime, unless the judge for good cause expressly authorizes execution at another time; and (iii) return the warrant to the magistrate judge designated in the warrant.

4. (U) **Warrant by Telephonic or Other Means**

(U) If a magistrate judge decides to proceed under FRCP Rule 41(d)(3)(A), the following additional procedures apply:

a. (U) **Preparing a Proposed Duplicate Original Warrant:** The applicant must prepare a "proposed duplicate original warrant" and must read or otherwise transmit the contents of that document verbatim to the magistrate judge.

b. (U) **Preparing an Original Warrant:** The magistrate judge must enter the contents of the proposed duplicate original warrant into an original warrant.

c. (U) **Modifications:** The magistrate judge may direct the applicant to modify the proposed duplicate original warrant. In that case, the judge must also modify the original warrant.

d. (U) **Signing the Original Warrant and the Duplicate Original Warrant:** Upon determining to issue the warrant, the magistrate judge must immediately sign the original warrant, enter on its face the exact time it is issued, and direct the applicant to sign the judge's name on the duplicate original warrant.

5. (U) **Executing and Returning the Warrant**

a. (U) **Noting the Time:** The officer executing the warrant must enter on its face the exact date and time it is executed.

b. (U) **Inventory:** An officer present during the execution of the warrant must prepare and verify an inventory of any property seized. The officer must do so in the presence of another officer and the person from whom, or from whose premises, the property was taken. If either one is not present, the officer must prepare and verify the inventory in the presence of at least one other credible person.

c. (U) **Receipt:** The officer executing the warrant must: (i) give a copy of the warrant and a receipt for the property taken to the person from whom, or from whose premises, the property was taken; or (ii) leave a copy of the warrant and receipt at the place where the officer took the property.

d. (U) **Return:** The officer executing the warrant must promptly return it — together with a copy of the inventory — to the magistrate judge designated on the warrant. The judge must, on request, give a copy of the inventory to the person from whom, or from whose premises, the property was taken and to the applicant for the warrant.

6. (U) **Forwarding Papers to the Clerk**

(U) The magistrate judge to whom the warrant is returned must attach to the warrant a copy of the return, the inventory, and all other related papers and must deliver them to the clerk in the district where the property was seized. (FRCP Rule 41)

7. (U) **Warrant for a Tracking Device**

a. (U) **Noting the time:** The officer executing a tracking device warrant must enter on it the exact date and time the device was installed and the period during which it was used.

b. (U) **Return:** Within 10 calendar days after the use of the tracking device has ended, the officer executing the warrant must return it to the judge designated in the warrant.

c. (U) **Service:** Within 10 calendar days after use of the tracking device has ended, the officer executing the warrant must serve a copy of the warrant on the person who was tracked. Service may be accomplished by delivering a copy to the person who, or whose property was tracked; or by leaving a copy at the person's residence or usual place of abode with an individual of suitable age and discretion who resides at that location and by mailing a copy to the person's last known address. Upon request of the government, the judge may delay notice as provided in FRCP Rule 41(f)(3).

8. (U) Delayed Notice

(U) Upon the government's request, a magistrate judge—or if authorized by FRCP Rule 41(b), a judge of a state court of record—may delay any notice required by FRCP Rule 41 if the delay is authorized by statute.

B. (U) Obtaining a FISA Warrant

(U) Applications for court-authorized physical search pursuant to FISA must be made by a federal officer in writing upon oath or affirmation and with the specific approval of the Attorney General. (See 50 U.S.C. § 1823) Each application must include:

1. (U) The identity of the federal officer making the application;

2. (U) The authority conferred on the Attorney General by the President and the approval of the Attorney General to make the application;

3. (U) The identity, if known, or description of the target of the physical search and a detailed description of the premises or property to be searched and of the information, material, or property to be seized, reproduced, or altered;

4. (U) A statement of the facts and circumstances relied upon and submitted by the applicant that there is probable cause to believe that:

   a. (U) The target is a foreign power or an agent of a foreign power, provided that no United States person may be considered a foreign power or an agent of a foreign power solely on the basis of activities protected by the First Amendment to the Constitution of the United States; and

   b. (U) Each of the facilities or places at which the FISA order is directed is being used by a foreign power or an agent of a foreign power.

5. (U) "In determining whether or not probable cause exists for purposes of an order under 50 U.S.C. § 1823(a)(3), a judge may consider past activities of the target, as well as facts and circumstances relating to current or future activities of the target." 50 U.S.C. § 1805(b). As it relates to United States citizens or aliens lawfully admitted for permanent residence, "agent of a foreign power" means any person who:

   a. (U) Knowingly engages in clandestine intelligence-gathering activities for or on behalf of a foreign power, whose activities involve or may involve a violation of the criminal statutes of the United States;

   b. (U) Pursuant to the direction of an intelligence service or network of a foreign power, knowingly engages in any other clandestine intelligence activities for or on behalf of such foreign power, whose activities involve or are about to involve a violation of the criminal statutes of the United States;

c. (U) Knowingly engages in sabotage or international terrorism, or activities that are in preparation therefore, for or on behalf of a foreign power;

d. (U) Knowingly enters the United States under a false or fraudulent identity for or on behalf of a foreign power or, while in the United States, knowingly assumes a false or fraudulent identity for or on behalf of a foreign power; or

e. (U) Knowingly aids or abets any person in the conduct of activities described in subparagraph 'a,' 'b,' or 'c,' above or knowingly conspires with any person to engage in activities described in subparagraph 'a,' 'b,' or 'c,' above. 50 U.S.C. § 1801(b) (2).

(U) For purposes of the above statute, 50 U.S.C. § 1801(a) (1) defines "foreign power" to include "a group engaged in international terrorism or activities in preparation therefore," 50 U.S.C. § 1801(a) (4), as well as, among other things, "a foreign government or any component thereof, whether or not recognized by the United States." Title 50 of the United States Code Section 1801(c) defines "international terrorism" as activities that:

(a) (U) Involve violent acts or acts dangerous to human life that are a violation of the criminal laws of the United States or of any State, or that would be a criminal violation if committed within the jurisdiction of the United States or any State;

(b) (U) Appear to be intended—

(1) (U) To intimidate or coerce a civilian population;

(2) (U) To influence the policy of a government by intimidation or coercion; or

(3) (U) To affect the conduct of a government by assassination or kidnapping; and

(c) (U) Occur totally outside the United States, or transcend national boundaries in terms of the means by which they are accomplished, the persons they appear intended to coerce or intimidate, or the locale in which their perpetrators operate or seek asylum by the applicant to justify the belief that: (i) the target is a foreign power or agent of a foreign power; (ii) the premises or property to be searched contains foreign intelligence information; and (iii) the premises or property to be searched is owned, used, possessed by, or is in transit to or from a foreign power or an agent of a foreign power.

6. (U) A statement of the proposed minimization procedures that have been approved by the Attorney General;

7. (U) A detailed description of the nature of the foreign intelligence information sought and the manner in which the physical search will be conducted;

8. (U) A Certification by the Director of the FBI or one of nine other individuals authorized by Congress or the President to provide such certifications that the information being sought is foreign intelligence information; that a significant purpose of the search is to obtain foreign intelligence information; that such information cannot reasonably be

obtained by normal investigative techniques; that the information sought is "foreign intelligence information" as defined by FISA; and includes a statement explaining the certifier's basis for the certification.

(U) **Note:** Title 50 of the United States Code Section 1804 specifies the Assistant to the President for National Security Affairs; E.O. 12949, as amended specifies the Director of the FBI, Deputy Director of the FBI, the Director of National Intelligence, the Principal Deputy Director of National Intelligence, the Director of the Central Intelligence Agency, the Secretary of State, the Deputy Secretary of State, the Secretary of Defense, and the Deputy Secretary of Defense as appropriate officials to make certifications required by FISA.

9. (U) Where the physical search may involve the residence of a United States person, the Attorney General must state what investigative techniques have previously been used to obtain the foreign intelligence information concerned and the degree to which these techniques resulted in acquiring such information;

10. (U) A statement of the facts concerning all previous applications before the FISA court that have been made involving any of the persons, premises, or property specified in the application and the actions taken on each previous application;

11. (U) The Attorney General may require any other affidavit or certification from any other officer in connection with an application; and

12. (U) The Court may require the applicant to furnish such other information as may be necessary to make the determinations required to issue an Order.

C. (U) **Length of Period of Authorization for FISC Orders**

1. (U) Generally, a FISC Order approving an unconsented physical search will specify the period of time during which physical searches are approved and provide that the government will be permitted the period of time necessary to achieve the purpose, or for 90 days, whichever is less, except that authority may be:

    a. (U) For no more than one year for "Foreign Power" targets (establishments); or

    b. (U) For no more than 120 days for an agent of a foreign power, with renewals for up to one year for non-United States persons.

2. (U) **An extension of physical search authority** may be granted on the same basis as the original order upon a separate application for an extension and upon new findings made in the same manner as the original order.

3. (U) **Emergency FISA Authority**

    a. (U) The Attorney General may authorize an emergency physical search under FISA when he reasonably makes a determination that an emergency situation exists that precludes advance FISA court review and approval, and there exists a factual predication for the issuance of a FISA Court Order. In such instances, a FISC judge must be informed by the Attorney General or his designee at the time of the authorization and an application according to FISA requirements is submitted to the judge as soon as is practicable but not more than seven (7) days after the emergency authority has been approved by the Attorney General.

b. (U) If a court order is denied after an emergency authorization has been initiated, no information gathered as a result of the search may be used in any manner except if with the approval of the Attorney General, the information indicates a threat of death or serious bodily harm to any person.

c. (U//FOUO) For an emergency FISA for physical search. [   ]

b2
b7E

4. (U) Special Circumstances

(U) The President through the Attorney General may also authorize a physical search under FISA without a court order for periods of up to one year, if the Attorney General certifies that the search will be solely directed at premises, information, material, or property that is used exclusively by or under the open and exclusive control of a foreign power; there is no substantial likelihood that the physical search will involve the premises, information, material, or property of a United States person; and there are minimization procedures that have been reported to the court and Congress. The FBI's involvement in such approvals is usually in furtherance of activities pursued according to E.O. 12333. Copies of such certifications are to be transmitted to the FISA Court (see 50 U.S.C. § 1822[a]).

(U) Information concerning United States persons acquired through unconsented physical searches may only be used according to minimization procedures. See: 50 U.S.C. §§ 1824(d)(4) and 1825(a).

5. (U) Required Notice

(U) If an authorized search involves the premises of a United States person, and the Attorney General determines that there is no national security interest in continuing the secrecy of the search, the Attorney General must provide notice to the United States person that the premises was searched and the identification of any property seized, altered, or reproduced during the search.

6. (U//FOUO) FISA Verification of Accuracy Procedures

(U//FOUO [   ]

b2
b7E

a. (U//FOUO) Each case file for which an application is prepared for submission to the FISC will include a sub-file to be labeled [   ] This sub-file is to contain copies of the supportive documentation relied upon when making the certifications to the [   ][   ] [   ] file is to include:

b2
b7E

i. (U//FOUO) [   ]

b2
b7E

ii. (U//FOUO) [   ]

b2
b7E

iii. (U//FOUO)

b2
b7E

b. (U//FOUO)

b2
b7E

7. (U//FOUO) **FISA Physical Search Administrative Sub-file**

(U//FOUO) Each case file for which an application is or has been prepared for submission to the FISC will include a sub-file to be labeled ⬚ This sub-file is to contain copies of all applications to and orders issued by the FISC for the conduct of physical searches in the investigative case. The following data must be included in this ⬚ ⬚ ⬚ ⬚.

b2
b7E

a. (U//FOUO)

b2
b7E

b. (U//FOUO)

b2
b7E

8. (U//FOUO) **FISA Review Board for FISA Renewals**

(U//FOUO)

b2
b7E

a. (U//FOUO)

b2
b7E

b. (U//FOUO)

b2
b7E

c. (U//FOUO)

b2
b7E

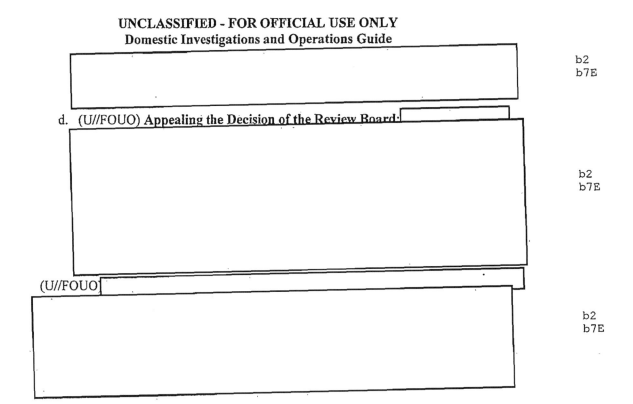

b2
b7E

d. (U//FOUO) **Appealing the Decision of the Review Board:**

b2
b7E

(U//FOUO)

b2
b7E

11.14. (U) Investigative Method: Acquisition of foreign intelligence information in conformity with Title VII of the Foreign Intelligence Surveillance Act

11.14.1. (U) Summary

(U) Titles I and III of the FISA (codified as 50 U.S.C. §§ 1801, et seq.) provide the standard, traditional methods of collection against agents of foreign powers (including United States and non-United States persons) and foreign power establishments inside the United States. Title VII of FISA, "Additional Procedures Regarding Certain Persons Outside the United States," provides means for collections of individuals outside the United States.

11.14.2. (U) Legal Authority

(U) FISA Amendments Act of 2008 (122 Stat 2436)

(U) AGG-Dom, Part V.A.13

11.14.3. (U) Definition of Investigative Method

(U) Title VII is to be used for conducting FISAs on certain persons located outside the United States

11.14.4. (U//FOUO) Standards for Use and Approval Requirements for Investigative Method

(U//FOUO) See requirements under DIOG Sections 11.12 and 11.13 and requirements specified above.

11.14.5. (U) Duration of Approval

(U//FOUO) See requirements under DIOG Sections 11.12 and 11.13

11.14.6. (U//FOUO) Specific Collection Procedures for Title VII

(U) The relevant procedures (or collections) under Title VII are:

A. **(U) Section 702 - "Procedures for Targeting Certain Persons Outside the United States Other than United States Persons"**

(U//FOUO) Under Section 702, the Government has the authority to target non-United States persons who are located outside the United States if the collection is effected with the assistance of a United States provider and if the collection occurs inside the United States. This section does not require a traditional FISA request. Rather, under this section the Attorney General and the Director of National Intelligence are required to file yearly determinations (filed as "Certifications") with the FISC that authorize the targeting of persons reasonably believed to be located outside the United States to acquire foreign intelligence information. The Certifications are accompanied by, in the case of the FBI, an affidavit signed by the FBI Director. In addition, the FBI is required to file "Targeting Procedures" designed to ensure that the acquisition is limited to persons reasonably believed to be located outside the United States and "to prevent the intentional acquisition of any communications as to which the sender and all intended recipients are known at the time of the acquisition to be located in the United States." Finally, the FBI is also required to follow minimization procedures.

B. (U) Section 703 - "Certain Acquisitions Inside the United States Targeting United States Persons Outside the United States"

(U//FOUO) Under Section 703, the Government has the authority to target United States persons who are located outside the United States if the collection is effected with the assistance of a United States provider and if the collection occurs inside the United States. This section only authorizes electronic surveillance or the acquisition of stored electronic communications or stored electronic data that requires a court order. Under this section, the FBI will submit a FISA request and obtain a FISC order and secondary orders, as needed. The process is the same as the current FISA process. Refer to the FISA Unit's website for further information. This section allows for emergency authorization and the FBI's Standard Minimization Procedures apply to the collection. Finally, under the statute, the surveillance must cease immediately if the target enters the United States. If the FBI wishes to surveil the United States person while he or she is in the United States, the FBI must obtain a separate court order under Title I (electronic surveillance) and/or Title III (physical search) of FISA in order to surveil that United States person while the person is located in the United States.

C. (U) Section 704 - "Other Acquisitions Targeting United States Persons Outside the United States"

(U//FOUO) Under Section 704, the Government has the authority to target United States persons who are located outside the United States if the collection occurs outside the United States (i.e., without the assistance of a United States' provider). The statute requires that the FISA court issue an order finding probable cause to believe that the United States person target is an agent of a foreign power and reasonably believed to be located outside the United States "under circumstances in which the targeted United States person has a reasonable expectation of privacy and a warrant would be required if the acquisition were conducted in the United States for law enforcement purposes." Under this section, the FBI will submit a FISA request and obtain a FISC order but will not obtain secondary orders. The process for obtaining these orders is the same as the current FISA request process. Refer to the FISA Unit's intranet website for further information. This section allows for emergency authorization and the FBI's Standard Minimization Procedures apply to the collection. Finally, surveillance authorized under this section must cease if the United States person enters the United States but may be re-started if the person is again reasonably believed to be outside the United States during the authorized period of surveillance. However, if there is a need to surveil the target while the target is located inside the United States, a separate court order must be obtained.

(U//FOUO) Generally, the FBI requires the assistance of other USIC agencies to implement this type of surveillance. Specific procedures for requesting that another USIC agency implement the surveillance for the FBI, if necessary, are classified and delineated in FBI Corporate Policy 121N.

D. (U) Section 705 - "Joint Applications and Concurrent Authorizations"

(U//FOUO) Section 705(a), "joint applications," allows for the FISC to, upon request of the FBI, authorize a joint application for targeting a United States person under both Sections 703 and 704 (inside and outside the United States simultaneously).

(U//FOUO) Section 705(b), "concurrent authorizations," states that if an order has been obtained under Section 105 (electronic surveillance under Title I of FISA) or 304 (physical search under Title III of FISA), the Attorney General may authorize the targeting of a United States person while such person is reasonably believed to be located outside the United States. The Attorney General has this authority under E.O. 12333 § 2.5. In other words, if a United States person target of a "regular" FISA travels outside the United States during the authorized period of the surveillance, the Attorney General, under Section 705(b) and E.O. 12333 § 2.5, can concurrently authorize surveillance to continue while the person is overseas obviating the need to obtain a separate order under Sections 703 or 704. To effectuate this authority, the Attorney General's "Approval page" on all FBI United States person FISAs contains standard language authorizing surveillance abroad, if needed.

(U//FOUO)

b2
b7E

12. (U) Assistance to Other Agencies

12.1. (U) Overview

(U//FOUO) Part II of the AGG-Dom authorizes the FBI to conduct investigations in order to detect or obtain information about, and prevent and protect against, federal crimes and threats to the national security and to collect foreign intelligence. Part III of the AGG-Dom, Assistance to Other Agencies, authorizes the FBI to provide investigative assistance to other federal, state, local or tribal, or foreign agencies when the investigation has those same objectives or when the investigative assistance is legally authorized for other purposes. Accordingly, FBI employees may provide assistance even if it is not for one of the purposes identified as grounds for an FBI investigation or assessment, if providing the assistance is otherwise authorized by law. For example, investigative assistance is legally authorized in certain contexts to state or local agencies in the investigation of crimes under state or local law, as provided in 28 U.S.C. §§ 540—felonious killing of state and local law enforcement officer; 540A—violent crime against travelers; 540B—serial killings, and to foreign agencies in the investigation of foreign law violations pursuant to international agreements. The FBI may use appropriate lawful methods in any authorized investigative assistance activity.

12.2. (U) Purpose and Scope

(U) The AGG-Dom permits FBI personnel to provide investigative assistance to:

A. (U) Authorized intelligence activities of other USIC agencies;

B. (U) Any federal agency in the investigation of federal crimes, threats to the national security, foreign intelligence collection, or any other purpose that may be lawfully authorized;

C. (U) Assist the President in determining whether to use the armed forces pursuant to 10 U.S.C. §§ 331-33, when DOJ-authorized as described in Section 12.5.B.1.c, below;

D. (U) Collect information necessary to facilitate public demonstrations in order to protect the exercise of First Amendment rights and ensure public health and safety, when DOJ-authorized and within the restrictions described in Section 12.5.B.1.d, below;

E. (U) State or local agencies in the investigation of crimes under state or local law where authorized by federal law (e.g., 28 U.S.C. §§ 540—felonious killing of state and local law enforcement officer; 540A—violent crime against travelers; 540B—serial killings);

F. (U) State, local, or tribal agencies in the investigation of matters that may involve federal crimes or threats to national security, or for such other purposes as may be legally authorized; and

G. (U) Foreign agencies in the investigations of foreign law violations pursuant to international agreements, and as otherwise set forth below, consistent with the interests of the United States (including national security interests) and with due consideration of the effect on any United States person.

(U) The FBI is further authorized to provide technical and scientific assistance to all duly constituted law enforcement agencies, other organizational units of the Department of Justice, and other federal agencies. 28 C.F.R. § 0.85(g). The FBI's authority and procedures for providing technical assistance is further set forth in Section 12.6 below.

(U) Authorized investigative assistance by the FBI to other agencies includes participation in joint operations and activities with such agencies. (AGG-Dom, Part III.E.1) The procedures for providing investigative assistance, together with the approval and notification requirements, are provided below.

12.3. (U//FOUO) Standards for Providing and Approving Investigative Assistance to Other Agencies

(U//FOUO) The determination of whether to provide FBI assistance to other agencies is both statutory and discretionary and must be based on consideration of the following factors:

A. (U//FOUO) Assistance is within the scope authorized by the AGG-Dom;

B. (U//FOUO) Assistance is not based solely on the exercise of First Amendment activities or on the race, ethnicity, national origin or religion of the subject; and

C. (U//FOUO) Assistance is an appropriate use of personnel and financial resources.

12.4. (U) Documentation, Record Retention and Dissemination

A. (U) **Documentation**

(U//FOUO) When providing assistance to a domestic or foreign agency, the required documentation in an appropriate case file includes: (i) the name and type of agency; (ii) the investigative methods used; (iii) the opening and closing dates of the request; and (iv) notifications required for the investigative activity.

b2
b7E

B. (U) **Records Retention for Assistance Furnished to Another Agency**

(U//FOUO) A database of records created with the [   ] is maintained to permit the prompt retrieval of the status of the assistance activity (opened or closed), the dates of opening and closing, and the basis for the assistance activity. (AGG-Dom, Part III.E.3)

b2
b7E

C. (U) **Dissemination of Information**

(U//FOUO) For unclassified information, the [   ] should be used to document the dissemination of information to: (i) United States Intelligence Community Agencies; (ii) United States Federal Agencies; (iii) State, Local, or Tribal Agencies; and (iv) Foreign Agencies. Dissemination to Foreign Agencies must be in accordance with the FBI Foreign Dissemination Manual, dated May 23, 2008. Classified information must be disseminated pursuant to applicable federal law, Presidential directive, Attorney General policy and FBI policy.

b2
b7E

12.5. (U) Duration, Approval and Notice for Investigative Assistance to Other Agencies

(U//FOUO) Investigative assistance that may be furnished to other agencies is described below by agency type. Dissemination of information to other agencies must be consistent with Director of National Intelligence directives, the AGG-Dom, DIOG Section 14, FBI Foreign Dissemination Manual, and any applicable MOU/MOA, law, treaty or other policy.

(U//FOUO) **Sensitive Investigative Matter:** Any assistance to other agencies involving a sensitive investigative matter requires CDC review, SAC approval, and notification to the appropriate FBIHQ substantive Unit Chief and Section Chief. (If assistance is to a foreign agency, notification to the Office of International Operations (OIO) Unit Chief and Section Chief is also required.) Additionally, FBIHQ must provide notice to the DOJ Criminal Division or NSD as soon as practicable, but not later than 30 calendar days after the initiation of any assistance involving a sensitive investigative matter (see classified appendix for additional notice requirements).

A. (U) **United States Intelligence Community Agencies**

1. (U) **Authority**

   (U//FOUO) The FBI may provide investigative assistance (including operational support) to authorized intelligence activities of other USIC agencies. (AGG-Dom, Part III.A) Investigative assistance must be in compliance with interagency memoranda of understanding/agreement, if applicable. For example, specific approval and notification requirements exist for CIA domestic activities.

2. (U) **Approval**

   (U//FOUO) Prior SSA approval is required for providing assistance to the USIC when the assistance uses investigative methods beyond those authorized in assessments. Assistance to other agencies using an investigative method authorized only for predicated investigations requires supervisory approval at the same level required for the respective investigative method if used in an FBI investigation. Specifically, higher supervisory approval and notification requirements may exist for conducting a joint operation (e.g., investigative operations with the Department of Defense [DoD], Department of Homeland Security), a sensitive investigative matter, and using particular investigative methods as noted in Sections 10 and 11, and the Division policy guides. Assistance for investigative methods beyond those authorized in assessments must be documented in the FD-999. Approval for use of specific technologies is set forth in Section 12.6 below and the OTD Manual.

B. (U) **United States Federal Agencies**

1. (U) **Authorities**

   a. (U//FOUO) The FBI may provide assistance to any other federal agency in the investigation of federal crimes or threats to the national security or in the collection of positive foreign intelligence. (Pursuant to Section 9, collection of positive foreign intelligence requires prior approval from FBIHQ CMS.) The FBI may provide investigative assistance to any federal agency for any other purpose that may be legally authorized, including investigative assistance to the Secret Service in support of its protective responsibilities. (AGG-Dom, Part III.B.1) See DIOG Section 12.6 below for guidance in providing technical assistance to federal agencies.

b. (U//FOUO) The FBI must follow MOU/MOA with other federal agencies where applicable. Specific approval and notification requirements exist for CIA and DoD domestic activities.

c. (U) **Actual or Threatened Domestic Civil Disorders**

   i. (U) At the direction of the Attorney General, the Deputy Attorney General, or the Assistant Attorney General for the Criminal Division, the FBI shall collect information relating to actual or threatened civil disorders to assist the President in determining (pursuant to the authority of the President under 10 U.S.C. §§ 331-33) whether use of the armed forces or militia is required and how a decision to commit troops should be implemented. The information sought shall concern such matters as: (AGG-Dom, Part III.B.2)

   (a) (U) The size of the actual or threatened disorder, both in number of people involved or affected and in a geographic area;

   (b) (U) The potential for violence;

   (c) (U) The potential for expansion of the disorder in light of community conditions and underlying causes of the disorder;

   (d) (U) The relationship of the actual or threatened disorder to the enforcement of federal law or court orders and the likelihood that state or local authorities will assist in enforcing those laws or orders; and

   (e) (U) The extent of state or local resources available to handle the disorder.

   ii. (U) Civil disorder investigations will be authorized only for a period of 30 days, but the authorization may be renewed for subsequent 30 day periods.

   iii. (U) The only investigative methods that may be used during a civil disorder investigation are:

   (a) (U) Obtain publicly available information;

   (b) (U) Access and examine FBI and other DOJ records, and obtain information from any FBI or other DOJ personnel;

   (c) (U) Access and examine records maintained by, and request information from, other federal, state, local, or tribal, or foreign governmental entities or agencies;

   (d) (U) Use online services and resources (whether nonprofit or commercial);

   (e) (U) Interview members of the public and private entities; and

   (U//FOUO) **Note:** Such interviews may only be conducted if the FBI employee identifies himself or herself as an FBI employee and accurately discloses the purpose of the interview.

   (f) (U) Accept information voluntarily provided by governmental or private entities.

(U) Other methods may be used only if authorized by the Attorney General, the Deputy Attorney General, or the Assistant Attorney General for the Criminal Division.

d. (U) **Public Health and Safety Authorities in Relation to Demonstrations**

i. (U) At the direction of the Attorney General, the Deputy Attorney General, or the Assistant Attorney General for the Criminal Division, the FBI shall collect information relating to demonstration activities that are likely to require the federal government to take action to facilitate the activities and provide public health and safety measures with respect to those activities. The information sought in such an investigation shall be that needed to facilitate an adequate federal response to ensure public health and safety and to protect the exercise of First Amendment rights, such as:

(a) (U) The time, place, and type of activities planned.

(b) (U) The number of persons expected to participate.

(c) (U) The expected means and routes of travel for participants and expected time of arrival.

(d) (U) Any plans for lodging or housing of participants in connection with the demonstration.

ii. (U) The only investigative methods that may be used in an investigation under this paragraph are:

(a) (U) Obtain publicly available information;

(b) (U) Access and examine FBI and other DOJ records, and obtain information from any FBI or other DOJ personnel;

(c) (U) Access and examine records maintained by, and request information from, other federal, state, local, or tribal, or foreign governmental entities or agencies;

(d) (U) Use online services and resources (whether nonprofit or commercial);

(e) (U) Interview of members of the public and private entities; and

(U//FOUO) **Note:** Such interviews may only be conducted if the FBI employee identifies himself or herself as an FBI employee and accurately discloses the purpose of the interview.

(f) (U) Accept information voluntarily provided by governmental or private entities.

(U) Other methods may be used only if authorized by the Attorney General, the Deputy Attorney General, or the Assistant Attorney General for the Criminal Division.

2. (U) **Approval**

(U//FOUO) Prior SSA approval is required for assistance to another federal agency when the assistance uses investigative methods beyond those authorized in assessments.

Assistance to other agencies using an investigative method authorized only for predicated investigations requires supervisory approval at the same level required for the respective investigative method if used in an FBI investigation, as provided in Section 11. Specifically, higher supervisory approval and notification requirements may exist for conducting a joint operation, a sensitive investigative matter, and using particular investigative methods, as noted in Sections 10 and 11 and in the Division policy guides. Assistance for investigative methods beyond those authorized in assessments must be documented in the FD-999. Approval for use of specific technologies is set forth in Section 12.6, below and the OTD Manual.

C. (U) **State, Local, or Tribal Agencies**

1. (U) **Authorities**

   a. (U) The FBI may provide investigative assistance to state, local, or tribal agencies in the investigation of matters that may involve federal crimes or threats to the national security, or for other legally authorized purposes. Legally authorized purposes include, but are not limited to, a specific federal statutory grant of authority such as that provided by 28 U.S.C. §§ 540—felonious killing of state and local law enforcement officer; 540A—violent crime against travelers; 540B—serial killings. (AGG-Dom, Part III.C) The FBI is further authorized to provide other material, scientific and technical assistance to state, local, and tribal agencies. (See 28 C.F.R. § 0.85[g] and DIOG Section 12.6, below.)

   b. (U//FOUO) The FBI must follow applicable MOU/MOA and/or treaties when it provides assistance to state, local, and tribal agencies.

   c. (U//FOUO) As a federal agency, the FBI's authority to investigate criminal offenses derives from federal statutes and is generally limited to violations of federal law. See 18 U.S.C. § 3052, 28 U.S.C. § 533 (1) and 28 C.F.R. § 0.85. With limited exceptions, such as those cited in Section 12.2.E., above, the FBI does not have any federal authority to investigate state crimes. FBI employees can assist in the investigation of other criminal matters with state and local authorities only if there is a reasonable basis to believe that the investigation will prevent, detect or lead to evidence of a violation of federal law or a threat to the national security.

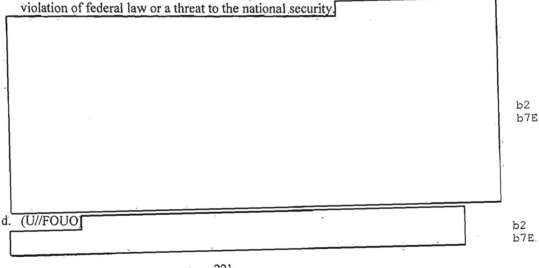

   d. (U//FOUO)

b2
b7E

b2
b7E

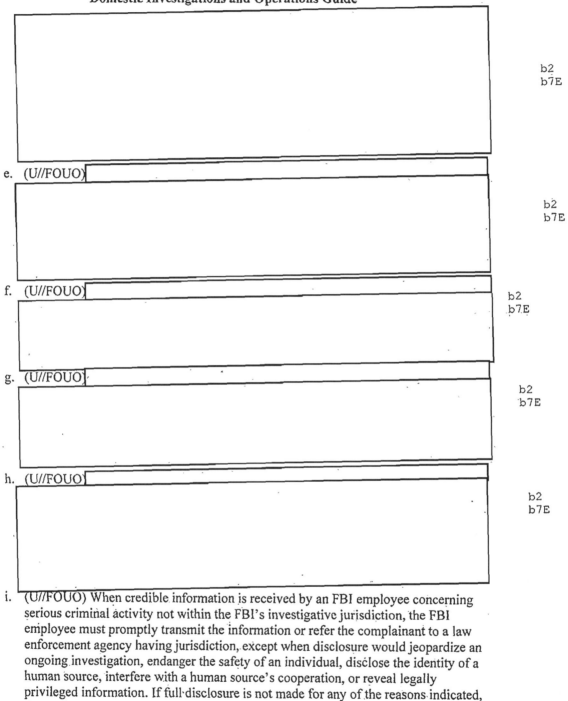

b2
b7E

b2
b7E

e. (U//FOUO)

b2
b7E

f. (U//FOUO)

b2
b7E

g. (U//FOUO)

b2
b7E

h. (U//FOUO)

b2
b7E

i. (U//FOUO) When credible information is received by an FBI employee concerning serious criminal activity not within the FBI's investigative jurisdiction, the FBI employee must promptly transmit the information or refer the complainant to a law enforcement agency having jurisdiction, except when disclosure would jeopardize an ongoing investigation, endanger the safety of an individual, disclose the identity of a human source, interfere with a human source's cooperation, or reveal legally privileged information. If full disclosure is not made for any of the reasons indicated, then, whenever feasible, the FBI employee must make at least limited disclosure to a law enforcement agency or agencies having jurisdiction, and full disclosure must be made as soon as the need for restricting the information is no longer present. Where disclosure is not made to the appropriate law enforcement agencies within 180 days, the FBI employee/Field Office must notify the appropriate substantive Unit at FBI Headquarters in writing concerning the facts and circumstances concerning the criminal activity. FBI Headquarters is required to make periodic reports to the Deputy Attorney General on such non-disclosure and incomplete disclosures. (AGG-Dom, Part VI.C.2)

2. (U) **Approval**

(U//FOUO) Prior SSA approval is required for assistance to state, local, or tribal agencies when the assistance uses investigative methods beyond those authorized in assessments. Assistance to other agencies using an investigative method authorized only for predicated investigations requires supervisory approval at the same level required for the respective investigative method if used in an FBI investigation. Specifically, higher supervisory approval and notification requirements may exist for conducting a joint operation, a sensitive investigative matter, and using particular investigative methods, as noted in Sections 10 and 11 and in the Division policy guides. Assistance for investigative methods beyond those authorized in assessments must be documented in the FD-999. Approval for use of specific technologies is set forth in Section 12.6, below and the OTD Manual.

D. (U) **Foreign Agencies**

1. (U//FOUO) **General:** The foundation of the FBI's international program is the Legat. Each Legat is the Director's personal representative in the foreign countries in which he/she resides or has regional responsibilities. The Legat's job is to respond to the FBI's domestic and foreign investigative needs. The Legat can accomplish this because he or she has developed partnerships and fostered cooperation with his or her foreign counterparts on every level and is familiar with investigative rules, protocols, and practices that differ from country to country. This is the Legat's primary responsibility. As such, foreign agency requests for assistance will likely come to the FBI through the Legat. If, however, foreign agency requests for assistance bypass the Legat, the FBI employee must notify the Legat and OIO, as discussed in greater detail below.

2. (U) **Authorities**

   a. (U//FOUO) At the request of foreign law enforcement, intelligence, or security agencies, the FBI may conduct investigations or provide assistance to investigations by such agencies, consistent with the interests of the United States (including national security interests) and with due consideration of the effect on any United States person. (AGG-Dom, Part III.D.1) The FBI must follow applicable MOUs, MOAs, Mutual Legal Assistance Treaties (MLAT) and other treaties when it provides assistance to foreign governments.

      i. (U//FOUO)

b2
b7E

ii. (U//FOUO)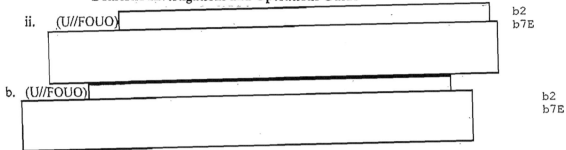

b2
b7E

b. (U//FOUO)

b2
b7E

c. (U//FOUO) The FBI may not provide assistance to foreign law enforcement, intelligence, or security officers conducting investigations within the United States unless such officers have provided prior written notification to the Attorney General of their status as an agent of a foreign government, as required by 18 U.S.C. § 951. (AGG-Dom, Part III.D.2) The notification required by 18 U.S.C. § 951 is not applicable to diplomats, consular officers or attachés.

d. (U//FOUO) Upon the request of a foreign government agency, the FBI may conduct background inquiries concerning individuals whose consent is documented. (AGG-Dom, Part III.D.3)

e. (U//FOUO) The AGG-Dom, Part III.D.4 authorizes the FBI to provide other material and technical assistance to foreign governments to the extent not otherwise prohibited by law. AG Order 2954-2008 authorizes the FBI to provide technical assistance to foreign governments, as referenced below in Section 12.6.

3. (U) **Approval**

a. (U//FOUO) Prior SSA approval is required for all assistance to foreign agencies. All assistance must be documented in the FD-999 and that approval should be documented in the file.

b. (U//FOUO)

c. (U//FOUO)

d. (U//FOUO)

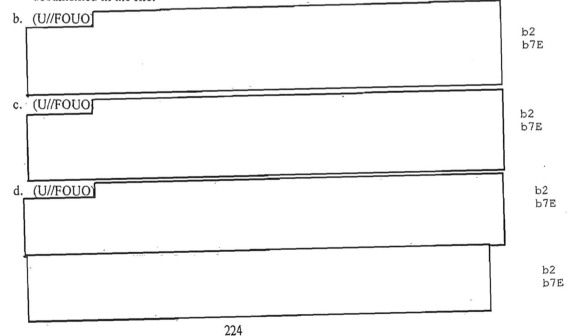

b2
b7E

b2
b7E

b2
b7E

b2
b7E

ii.   (U//FOUO) [REDACTED]

    b2
    b7E

4. (U) **Notice**

   a. (U//FOUO) [REDACTED]

    b2
    b7E

   b. (U) The FBI must notify the DOJ NSD concerning investigation or assistance where both: (i) FBIHQs approval for the activity is required (e.g., FBIHQ approval required to use a particular investigative method); and (ii) the activity relates to a threat to the United States national security. The FBIHQ Division approving the use of the investigative method must notify DOJ NSD as soon as practicable, but no later than 30 calendar days after FBIHQ approval (see classified appendix for [REDACTED] [REDACTED]. (AGG-Dom, Part III.D.1)

    b2
    b7E

5. (U) **Dissemination**

(U//FOUO) All dissemination of FBI information to foreign agencies must be conducted according to the FBI Foreign Dissemination Manual, dated May 23, 2008

12.6. (U//FOUO) **Standards for Providing and Approving Technical Assistance to Foreign, State, Local and Tribal Agencies**

A. (U) **Authority**

   1. (U//FOUO) [REDACTED]

    b2
    b7E

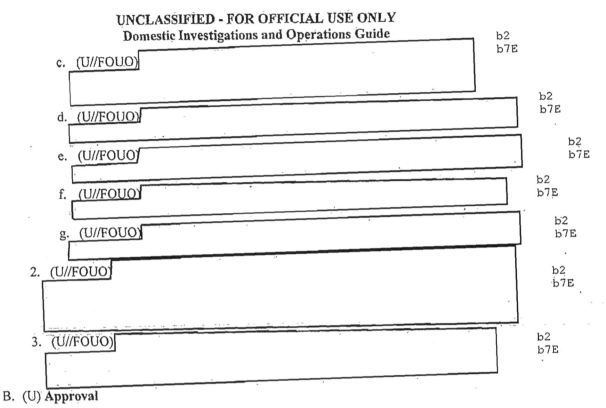

c. (U//FOUO)   b2
                                                                               b7E

d. (U//FOUO)   b2
                                                                               b7E

e. (U//FOUO)   b2
                                                                               b7E

f. (U//FOUO)   b2
                                                                               b7E

g. (U//FOUO)   b2
                                                                               b7E

2. (U//FOUO)   b2
                                                                               b7E

3. (U//FOUO)   b2
                                                                               b7E

B. (U) **Approval**

(U//FOUO) All technical assistance must be approved by the Director or his designated senior executive FBI official, as provided in the OTD manual. All technical assistance must be documented in an FBI assessment file, predicated investigation file, a domestic police cooperation file, a foreign police cooperation file, or other investigative/technical assistance control file. Additionally, all technical assistance must be documented in the FD-999 or its successor.

13. (U) Extraterritorial Provisions

13.1. (U) Overview

(U//FOUO) The FBI may conduct investigations abroad, participate with foreign officials in investigations abroad, or otherwise conduct activities outside the United States. The guidelines for conducting investigative activities outside of the United States are currently contained in: (i) *The Attorney General's Guidelines for Extraterritorial FBI Operations and Criminal Investigations*; (ii) *The Attorney General's Guidelines for FBI National Security Investigations and Foreign Intelligence Collection*; and (iii) *The Attorney General Guidelines on the Development and Operation of FBI Criminal Informants and Cooperative Witnesses in Extraterritorial Jurisdictions* (collectively, the Extraterritorial Guidelines). The *Attorney General's Guidelines for Extraterritorial FBI Operations* are currently being drafted, as discussed in DIOG Section 2.1, and will supercede the above listed guidelines, or applicable provisions thereof.

13.2. (U) Purpose and Scope

(U//FOUO) As a general rule, the Extraterritorial Guidelines apply when FBI personnel or confidential human sources are actively engaged in investigative activity outside the borders of the United States.

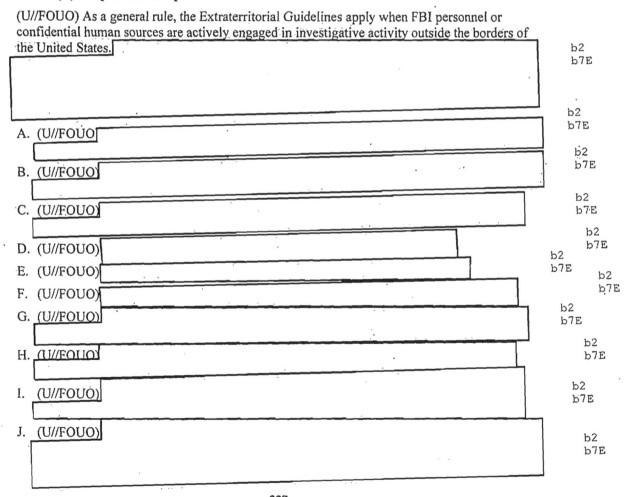

A. (U//FOUO)

B. (U//FOUO)

C. (U//FOUO)

D. (U//FOUO)

E. (U//FOUO)

F. (U//FOUO)

G. (U//FOUO)

H. (U//FOUO)

I. (U//FOUO)

J. (U//FOUO)

b2
b7E

(U//FOUO) FBI personnel planning to engage in any of the investigative activities described in the subsection above must obtain the concurrence of the appropriate Legat and must comply with the remaining procedural requirement of the Extraterritorial Guidelines. For additional information consult the Extraterritorial Section of the OGC website.

13.3. (U) Legal Attache Program

(U//FOUO) The foundation of the FBI's international program is the Legat. Each Legat is the Director's personal representative in the foreign countries in which he/she resides or has regional responsibilities. The Legat's job is to respond to the FBI's domestic and extraterritorial investigative needs. Legats can accomplish this mission because they have developed partnerships and fostered cooperation with their foreign counterparts on every level and are familiar with local investigative rules, protocols, and practices which differ from country to country. For additional information consult the FBIHQ OIO website.

14. (U) Retention and Sharing of Information

14.1. (U) Purpose and Scope

(U//FOUO) Every FBI component is responsible for the creation and maintenance of authentic, reliable, and trustworthy records. Without complete and accessible records, the FBI cannot conduct investigations, gather and analyze intelligence, assist with the prosecution of criminals, or perform any of its critical missions effectively.

(U//FOUO) The FBI is committed to ensuring that its records management program accomplishes the following goals:

A. (U//FOUO) Facilitates the documentation of official decisions, policies, activities, and transactions;

B. (U//FOUO) Facilitates the timely retrieval of needed information;

C. (U//FOUO) Ensures continuity of FBI business;

D. (U//FOUO) Controls the creation and growth of FBI records;

E. (U//FOUO) Reduces operating costs by managing records according to FBI business needs and by disposing of unneeded records in a timely manner;

F. (U//FOUO) Improves efficiency and productivity through effective records storage and retrieval methods;

G. (U//FOUO) Ensures compliance with applicable laws and regulations;

H. (U//FOUO) Safeguards the FBI's mission-critical information;

I. (U//FOUO) Preserves the FBI's corporate memory and history; and

J. (U//FOUO) Implements records management technologies to support all of the goals listed above.

14.2. (U) The FBI's Records Retention Plan, and Documentation

(U//FOUO) The FBI must retain records relating to investigative activities according to a records retention plan approved by the NARA. (AGG-Dom, Part VI.A.1)

(U//FOUO) The FBI's disposition authorities provide specific instructions about the length of time that records must be maintained. In some instances, records may be destroyed after a prescribed period of time has elapsed. Other records are never destroyed and are transferred to NARA a certain number of years after a case was closed.

A. (U//FOUO) The FBI must maintain a database or records system that permits, with respect to each predicated investigation, the prompt retrieval of the status of the investigation (open or closed), the dates of opening and closing, and the basis for the investigation. (AGG-Dom, Part VI.A.2)

(U//FOUO) The FBI has updated its official File Classification System to cover records related to all investigative and intelligence collection activities, including assessments. Records are maintained in the FBI's Central Records System or other designated systems of records, that provide the required maintenance and retrieval functionality.

B. (U//FOUO) Assessments must also adhere to the standards as set forth in the Records Management Division Disposition Plan and Retention Plan. All records, including assessments, may be destroyed or expunged earlier than the destruction schedule through proper authority.

(U//FOUO) All Bureau records are maintained for their full retention periods, except under certain circumstances under which they may be either destroyed earlier or retained longer. Records may be retained for a longer period than their disposition authority specifies, if they are subject to a litigation freeze. Court orders may direct that certain records be expunged from a case file, or (more rarely) that the entire case file be expunged. Under certain circumstances, individuals may also request that certain records be expunged. Expungement of records may mean the physical removal and destruction of some or all of the record or, depending on the court order and the governing statute or program, it may mean the removal, sealing, and secure storage of records away from the remaining file. In most instances, only certain documents, not the entire file, are subject to expungement.

14.3. (U) Information Sharing

(U//FOUO) The FBI 2008 National Information Sharing Strategy (NISS) provides the common vision, goals, and framework needed to guide information sharing initiatives with our federal, state, local, and tribal agency partners; foreign government counterparts, and private sector stakeholders. The FBI NISS addresses the cultural and technological changes required to move the FBI to "a responsibility to provide" culture. This will be accomplished by using the best practices and technology standards of both communities as we support the intelligence and law enforcement communities in collection, dissemination, analysis, collaboration, and operational efforts.

A. (U) Permissive Sharing

(U//FOUO) Consistent with the Privacy Act and any other applicable laws and memoranda of understanding or agreement with other agencies concerning the dissemination of information, the FBI may disseminate information obtained or produced through activities under the AGG-Dom:

1. (U//FOUO) Within the FBI and to all other components of the Department of Justice if the recipients have need of the information in the performance of their official duties.

2. (U//FOUO) To other federal agencies if disclosure is compatible with the purpose for which the information was collected and it is related to their responsibilities. In relation to other USIC agencies, the determination whether the information is related to the recipient responsibilities may be left to the recipient.

3. (U//FOUO) To state, local, or Indian tribal agencies directly engaged in the criminal justice process where access is directly related to a law enforcement function of the recipient agency.

4. (U//FOUO) To congressional committees as authorized by the DOJ Office of Legislative Affairs.

5. (U//FOUO) To foreign agencies if the FBI determines that the information is related to their responsibilities; the dissemination is consistent with the interests of the United

States (including national security interests); and where the purpose of the disclosure is compatible with the purpose for which the information was collected.

6. (U//FOUO) If the information is publicly available, does not identify United States persons, or is disseminated with the consent of the person whom it concerns.

7. (U//FOUO) If the dissemination is necessary to protect the safety or security of persons or property, to protect against or prevent a crime or imminent threat to the national security, or to obtain information for the conduct of an authorized FBI investigation.

8. (U//FOUO) If dissemination of the information is otherwise permitted by the Privacy Act (5 U.S.C.§ 552a) (AGG-Dom, Part VI.B.1)

(U//FOUO) All FBI information sharing activities under this section shall be according to Corporate Policy Directive 12D, "FBI Sharing Activities with Other Government Agencies," 95D "Protecting Privacy in the Information Sharing Environment," and any amendments thereto and applicable succeeding policy directives.

B. (U) **Required Sharing**

(U//FOUO) The FBI must share and disseminate information as required by statutes, treaties, Executive Orders, Presidential directives, National Security Council directives, Homeland Security Council directives, DNI directives, Attorney General-approved policies, and MOUs or MOAs, as consistent with the Privacy Act.

14.4. (U) Information Related to Criminal Matters

A. (U) **Coordinating with Prosecutors**

(U//FOUO) In an investigation relating to possible criminal activity in violation of federal law, the FBI employee conducting the investigation must maintain periodic written or oral contact with the appropriate federal prosecutor, as circumstances warrant and as requested by the prosecutor. When, during such an investigation, a matter appears arguably to warrant prosecution, the FBI employee must present the relevant facts to the appropriate federal prosecutor. Information on investigations that have been closed must be available on request to a United States Attorney or his or her designee or an appropriate Department of Justice official. (AGG-Dom, Part VI.C)

B. (U) **Criminal Matters Outside FBI Jurisdiction**

(U//FOUO) When credible information is received by an FBI employee concerning serious criminal activity not within the FBI's investigative jurisdiction, the FBI employee must promptly transmit the information or refer the complainant to a law enforcement agency having jurisdiction, except where disclosure would jeopardize an ongoing investigation, endanger the safety of an individual, disclose the identity of a CHS, interfere with the cooperation of a CHS, or reveal legally privileged information. If full disclosure is not made for the reasons indicated, then, whenever feasible, the FBI employee must make at least limited disclosure to a law enforcement agency or agencies having jurisdiction, and full disclosure must be made as soon as the need for restricting disclosure is no longer present. Where full disclosure is not made to the appropriate law enforcement agencies within 180 days, the FBI employee/Field Office must promptly notify FBIHQ in writing of the facts and circumstances concerning the criminal activity. The FBI must make periodic reports to the

Deputy Attorney General on such non-disclosures and incomplete disclosures, in a form suitable to protect the identity of a CHS. (AGG-Dom, Part VI.C)

C. (U) **Reporting of Criminal Activity**

(U//FOUO) When it appears that an FBI employee has engaged in criminal activity in the course of an investigation under the AGG-Dom, the FBI must notify the USAO or an appropriate DOJ Division. When it appears that a CHS has engaged in criminal activity in the course of an investigation under the AGG-Dom, the FBI must proceed as provided in the AGG-CHS. When information concerning possible criminal activity by any other person appears in the course of an investigation under the AGG-Dom, the FBI must initiate an investigation of the criminal activity if warranted. (AGG-Dom, Part VI.C.3)

(U//FOUO) The reporting requirements under this paragraph relating to criminal activity by an FBI employee or a CHS do not apply to otherwise illegal activity that is authorized in conformity with the AGG-Dom or other Attorney General guidelines or to minor traffic offenses. (AGG-Dom, Part VI.C.3)

14.5. (U) Information Related to National Security and Foreign Intelligence Matters

(U//FOUO) All information sharing with a foreign government related to classified national security and foreign intelligence must adhere to the FBI Foreign Dissemination Manual effective 05/23/2008 and effective policies governing MOUs.

(U//FOUO) The general principle reflected in current law and policy is that there is a responsibility to provide information as consistently and fully as possible to agencies with relevant responsibilities to protect the United States and its people from terrorism and other threats to the national security, except as limited by specific constraints on such sharing. The FBI's responsibility in this area includes carrying out the requirements of the MOU Between the Intelligence Community, Federal Law Enforcement Agencies, and the Department of Homeland Security Concerning Information Sharing (March 4, 2003), or any successor memorandum of understanding or agreement. Specific requirements also exist for internal coordination and consultation with other DOJ components, and for sharing national security and foreign intelligence information with White House agencies, as provided in the ensuing paragraphs. (AGG-Dom, Part VI.D)

(U) **Department of Justice**

A. (U//FOUO) The DOJ NSD must have access to all information obtained by the FBI through activities relating to threats to the national security or foreign intelligence. The Director of the FBI and the Assistant Attorney General for National Security must consult concerning these activities whenever requested by either of them, and the FBI must provide such reports and information concerning these activities as the Assistant Attorney General for National Security may request. In addition to any reports or information the Assistant Attorney General for National Security may specially request under this subparagraph, the FBI must provide annual reports to the NSD concerning its foreign intelligence collection program, including information concerning the scope and nature of foreign intelligence collection activities in each FBI Field Office. (AGG-Dom, Part VI.D.1)

B. (U//FOUO) The FBI must keep the NSD apprised of all information obtained through activities under the AGG-Dom that is necessary to the ability of the United States to investigate or protect against threats to the national security, that includes regular consultations between the FBI and the NSD to exchange advice and information relevant to addressing such threats through criminal prosecution or other means. (AGG-Dom, Part VI.D.1)

C. (U//FOUO) Except for counterintelligence investigations, a relevant USAO must have access to and must receive information from the FBI relating to threats to the national security, and may engage in consultations with the FBI relating to such threats, to the same extent as the NSD. The relevant USAO must receive such access and information from the FBI Field Offices. (AGG-Dom, Part VI.D.1)

D. (U//FOUO) In a counterintelligence investigation – e.g., an investigation relating to a matter described in Part VII.S.2 of the AGG-Dom – the FBI's providing information to and consultation with a relevant USAO is subject to authorization by the NSD. In consultation with the Executive Office for United States Attorneys and the FBI, the NSD must establish policies setting forth circumstances in which the FBI will consult with the NSD prior to informing a relevant USAO about such an investigation. The policies established by the NSD must (among other things) provide that:

1. (U//FOUO) The NSD will, within 30 days, authorize the FBI to share with the USAO information relating to certain espionage investigations, as defined by the policies, unless such information is withheld because of substantial national security considerations; and

2. (U//FOUO) The FBI may consult freely with the USAO concerning investigations within the scope of this subparagraph during an emergency, so long as the NSD is notified of such consultation as soon as practicable after the consultation. (AGG-Dom, Part VI.D.1)

E. (U//FOUO) Information shared with a USAO pursuant to DIOG subparagraph 14.5 (National Security) must be disclosed only to the United States Attorney or any AUSA designated by the United States Attorney as points of contact to receive such information. The United States Attorney and designated AUSA must have an appropriate security clearance and must receive training in the handling of classified information and information derived from FISA, including training concerning the secure handling and storage of such information and training concerning requirements and limitations relating to the use, retention, and dissemination of such information. (AGG-Dom, Part VI.D.1)

F. (U//FOUO) The disclosure and sharing of information by the FBI under this paragraph is subject to any limitations required in orders issued by the FISC, controls imposed by the originators of sensitive material, and restrictions established by the Attorney General or the Deputy Attorney General in particular cases. The disclosure and sharing of information by the FBI under this paragraph that may disclose the identity of a CHS is governed by the relevant provisions of the AGG-CHS. (AGG-Dom, Part VI.D.1)

(U) White House

(U//FOUO) In order to carry out their responsibilities, the President, the Vice President, the Assistant to the President for National Security Affairs, the Assistant to the President for Homeland Security Affairs, the National Security Council (NSC) and its staff, the Homeland Security Council (HSC) and its staff, and other White House officials and offices require information from all federal agencies, including foreign intelligence, and information relating to international terrorism and other threats to the national security. The FBI accordingly may disseminate to the White House foreign intelligence and national security information obtained through activities under the AGG-Dom, subject to the following standards and procedures.

A. (U//FOUO) White House must request such information through the NSC staff or HSC staff including, but not limited to, the NSC Legal and Intelligence Directorates and Office of Combating Terrorism, or through the President's Intelligence Advisory Board or the Counsel to the President. (AGG-Dom, Part VI.D.2.a)

    (U//FOUO) If the White House sends a request for such information to the FBI without first sending the request through the entities described above, the request must be returned to the White House for resubmission.

B. (U//FOUO) Compromising information concerning domestic officials or political organizations, or information concerning activities of United States persons intended to affect the political process in the United States, may be disseminated to the White House only with the approval of the Attorney General, based on a determination that such dissemination is needed for foreign intelligence purposes, for the purpose of protecting against international terrorism or other threats to the national security, or for the conduct of foreign affairs. However, such approval is not required for dissemination to the White House of information concerning efforts of foreign intelligence services to penetrate the White House, or concerning contacts by White House personnel with foreign intelligence service personnel. (AGG-Dom, Part VI.D.2.b)

C. (U//FOUO) Examples of types of information that are suitable for dissemination to the White House on a routine basis include, but are not limited to (AGG-Dom, Part VI.D.2.c):

    1. (U//FOUO) Information concerning international terrorism;

    2. (U//FOUO) Information concerning activities of foreign intelligence services in the United States;

    3. (U//FOUO) Information indicative of imminent hostilities involving any foreign power;

    4. (U//FOUO) Information concerning potential cyber threats to the United States or its allies;

    5. (U//FOUO) Information indicative of policy positions adopted by foreign officials, governments, or powers, or their reactions to United States foreign policy initiatives;

    6. (U//FOUO) Information relating to possible changes in leadership positions of foreign governments, parties, factions, or powers;

    7. (U//FOUO) Information concerning foreign economic or foreign political matters that might have national security ramifications; and

    8. (U//FOUO) Information set forth in regularly published national intelligence requirements.

D. (U//FOUO) Communications by the FBI to the White House that relate to a national security matter and concern a litigation issue for a specific pending case must be made known to the Office of the Attorney General, the Office of the Deputy Attorney General, or the Office of the Associate Attorney General. White House policy may limit or prescribe the White House personnel who may request information concerning such issues from the FBI. (AGG-Dom Part VI.D.2.d)

E. (U//FOUO) The limitations on dissemination of information by the FBI to the White House under the AGG-Dom do not apply to dissemination to the White House of information acquired in the course of an FBI investigation requested by the White House into the background of a potential employee or appointee, or responses to requests from the White House under E.O. 10450 relating to security requirements for government employment. (AGG-Dom, Part VI.D.2.e)

14.6. (U) Special Statutory Requirements

A. (U) <u>Dissemination</u> of information acquired under the FISA is, to the extent provided in that Act, subject to <u>minimization procedures</u> and other requirements specified in that Act. (AGG-Dom, Part VI.D.3.a)

B. (U) Information obtained through the use of NSLs under 15 U.S.C. § 1681v (NSLs to obtain full credit reports) may be disseminated in conformity with the general standards of AGG-Dom, Part VI, and DIOG <u>Section 11.9.3.G</u>. Information obtained through the use of NSLs under other statutes may be disseminated in conformity with the general standards of the AGG-Dom, Part VI, subject to any applicable limitations in their governing statutory provisions (see DIOG Section 11.9.3.G): 12 U.S.C. § 3414(a)(5)(B); 15 U.S.C. § 1681u(f); 18 U.S.C. § 2709(d); 50 U.S.C. § 436(e). (AGG-Dom, Part VI.D.3.b)

15. (U) Intelligence Analysis and Planning

15.1. (U) Overview

(U//FOUO) The AGG-Dom provide specific guidance and authorization for intelligence analysis and planning. This authority enables the FBI to identify and understand trends, causes, and potential indicia of criminal activity and other threats to the United States that would not be apparent from the investigation of discrete matters alone. By means of intelligence analysis and planning, the FBI can more effectively discover criminal threats, threats to the national security, and other matters of national intelligence interest, and can provide the critical support needed for the effective discharge of its investigative responsibilities and other authorized activities. (AGG-Dom, Part IV)

(U//FOUO) In carrying out its intelligence functions under Part IV of the AGG-Dom, the FBI is authorized to collect information using all assessment investigative methods authorized in Part II of the AGG-Dom as described in the DIOG Section 5.

b2
b7E

Investigative activities under the AGG-Dom and other legally authorized activities through which the FBI acquires information, data, or intelligence may properly be utilized, structured, and prioritized to support and effectuate the FBI's intelligence mission. (AGG-Dom, Part II.A.3.d and Part IV, Intro.)

(U//FOUO) **Note:** In the DIOG, the word "assessment" has two distinct meanings. The AGG-Dom authorizes as an investigative activity an "assessment," which requires an authorized purpose as discussed in Section 5. The USIC, however, also uses the word "assessment" to describe written intelligence products, as discussed in Section 15.7.B.

15.2. (U) Purpose and Scope

A. (U//FOUO) **Functions Authorized:** The AGG-Dom authorizes the FBI to engage in intelligence analysis and planning to facilitate and support investigative activities and other authorized activities. The functions authorized include:

1. (U//FOUO) Development of overviews and analyses concerning threats to and vulnerabilities of the United States and its interests, such as domain management as related to the FBI's responsibilities;

2. (U//FOUO) Research and analysis to produce reports and assessments (analytical products) concerning matters derived from or relevant to investigative activities or other authorized FBI activities; and

3. (U//FOUO) The operation of intelligence and information systems that facilitate and support investigations and analysis through the compilation and analysis of data and information on an ongoing basis. (AGG-Dom, Introduction B)

B. (U//FOUO) **Integration of Intelligence Activities:** In order to protect against national security and criminal threats through intelligence-driven operations, the FBI should integrate intelligence activities into all investigative efforts by:

1. (U//FOUO) Systematically assessing particular geographic areas or sectors to identify potential threats, vulnerabilities, gaps, and collection opportunities in response to FBI collection requirements that support the broad range of FBI responsibilities;

2. (U//FOUO) Pro-actively directing resources to collect against potential threats and other matters of interest to the nation and the FBI, and developing new collection capabilities where needed;

3. (U//FOUO) Continuously validating collection capabilities to ensure information integrity;

4. (U//FOUO) Deliberately gathering information in response to articulated priority intelligence requirements using all available collection resources, then expeditiously preparing the collected information for analysis and dissemination and promptly disseminating it to appropriate partners at the local, state, national and foreign level; and

5. (U//FOUO) Purposefully evaluating the implications of collected information on current and emerging threat issues.

C. (U//FOUO) **Analysis and Planning not Requiring the Initiation of an AGG-Dom Part II Assessment,** (see DIOG Section 5):

b2
b7E

As part of such analysis, an FBI employee can analyze historical information already contained within: (i) FBI data systems; (ii) USIC systems to which the FBI employee has access (e.g., _____); (iii) any other United States Government data system to which the FBI employee has access; and (iv) the FBI employee can also conduct open-source Internet searches. Open-source Internet searches do not include any paid-for-service databases such as Lexis-Nexis and Choicepoint.

b2
b7E

b2
b7E

15.3. (U) Civil Liberties and Privacy

(U) The FBI must collect intelligence critical to the FBI's ability to carry out its intelligence and law enforcement mission. While conducting intelligence analysis and planning, the FBI will conduct its activities in compliance with the Constitution, federal laws, the AGG-Dom and other relevant authorities in order to protect civil liberties and privacy.

15.4. (U) Legal Authority

(U) The FBI is an intelligence agency as well as a law enforcement agency. Accordingly, its basic functions extend beyond limited investigations of discrete matters, and include broader analytic and planning functions. The FBI's responsibilities in this area derive from various administrative and statutory sources. See, e.g., E.O. 12333 § 1.7(g); 28 U.S.C. §§ 532 note (incorporating P.L. 108-458 §§ 2001-2003) and 534 note (incorporating P.L. 109-162 § 1107).

(U//FOUO) The scope of authorized activities under Part II of the AGG-Dom is not limited to "investigation" in a narrow sense, such as solving particular cases or obtaining evidence for use in particular criminal prosecutions. Rather, the investigative activities authorized under the AGG-Dom may be properly used to provide critical information needed for broader analytic and intelligence purposes to facilitate the solution and prevention of crime, protect the national security, and further foreign intelligence objectives. These purposes include use of the information in intelligence analysis and planning under AGG-Dom, Part IV, and dissemination of the information to other law enforcement, USIC, and White House agencies under AGG-Dom, Part VI. Accordingly, information obtained at all stages of investigative activity is to be retained and disseminated for these purposes as provided in the AGG-Dom, or in FBI policy consistent with the AGG-Dom, regardless of whether it furthers investigative objectives in a narrower or more immediate sense. (AGG-Dom, Part II)

15.5. (U//FOUO) Standards for Initiating or Approving Intelligence Analysis and Planning

(U//FOUO) If an FBI employee wishes to engage in Intelligence Analysis and Planning that requires the collection or examination of information not available: (i) through an open-source Internet search; (ii) in the FBI's existing files; (iii) in the USIC data systems to which the FBI employee has access; or (iv) in any other United States Government data system to which the FBI employee has acces, an assessment must be initiated. An FBI employee or approving official must determine that:

A. (U//FOUO) An authorized purpose and objective exists for the conduct of an assessment (e.g., information is needed in order to conduct appropriate intelligence analysis and planning);

B. (U//FOUO) The assessment is based on factors other than the exercise of First Amendment activities or on the race, ethnicity, national origin or religion of the subject; and

C. (U//FOUO) The assessment is an appropriate use of personnel and financial resources.

15.6. (U//FOUO) Standards for Initiating or Approving the Use of an Authorized Investigative Method in Intelligence Analysis and Planning

A. (U//FOUO) The use of the particular investigative method is likely to further an objective of the assessment;

B. (U//FOUO) The investigative method selected is the least intrusive method, reasonable under the circumstances;

C. (U//FOUO) If the assessment relates to positive foreign intelligence, the FBI must operate openly and consensually with United States persons, to the extent practicable.

D. (U//FOUO) The anticipated value of the assessment justifies the use of the selected investigative method or methods; and

E. (U//FOUO) The investigative method is an appropriate use of personnel and financial resources.

15.7. (U) Authorized Activities in Intelligence Analysis and Planning

(U) The FBI may engage in intelligence analysis and planning to facilitate or support investigative activities authorized by the AGG-Dom or other legally authorized activities. Activities the FBI may carry out as part of Intelligence Analysis and Planning include:

A. (U//FOUO) **Strategic Intelligence Analysis**

(U//FOUO) The FBI is authorized to develop overviews and analyses of threats to and vulnerabilities of the United States and its interests in areas related to the FBI's responsibilities, including domestic and international criminal threats and activities; domestic and international activities, circumstances, and developments affecting the national security. FBI overviews and analyses may encompass present, emergent, and potential threats and vulnerabilities, their contexts and causes, and identification and analysis of means of responding to them. (AGG-Dom, Part IV)

1. (U//FOUO) **Domain Management by Field Offices**

(U//FOUO) As part of Strategic Analysis Planning activities, the FBI may collect information in order to improve or facilitate "domain awareness" and may engage in "domain management." "Domain management" is the systematic process by which the FBI develops cross-programmatic domain awareness and leverages its knowledge to enhance its ability to: (i) proactively identify threats, vulnerabilities, and intelligence gaps; (ii) discover new opportunities for needed intelligence collection and prosecution; and (iii) set tripwires to provide advance warning of national security and criminal threats. Effective domain management enables the FBI to identify significant threats, detect vulnerabilities within its local and national domain, identify new sources and threat indicators, and recognize new trends so that resources can be appropriately allocated at the local level in accordance with national priorities.

(U//FOUO) Through a properly authorized assessment, domain management is undertaken at the local and national levels. All National Domain Assessments are initiated and coordinated by the DI. Examples of domain management activities include, but are not limited to: [   ] census crime statistics, case information, domain entities, trend analysis, source development, and placement of tripwires. Further guidance regarding domain management and examples of intelligence products are contained in the [   ]

b2
b7E

(U//FOUO) The Field Office "domain" is the territory and issues for which a Field Office exercises responsibility, also known as the Field Office's area-of-responsibility (AOR). Domain awareness is the: (i) strategic understanding of national security and criminal threats and vulnerabilities; (ii) FBI's positioning to collect against these threats and vulnerabilities; and (iii) the existence of intelligence gaps related to the domain.

(U//FOUO) All information collected for domain management must be documented in an [   ] as directed in the [   ]

b2
b7E

[   ]. Additionally, at any time that [   ] a separate substantive classification assessment file or subfile, according to the investigative matter, must be opened on the individual.

FBIHQ DI provides specific guidance in its [   ] regarding, but not limited to: the initiation, opening, coordination and purpose for Field Office and National Domain Assessments.

b2
b7E

2. (U//FOUO) **Collection Management**

(U//FOUO) Collection Management is a formal business process through which Intelligence Information Needs and Intelligence Gaps (e.g., unknowns) are expressed as Intelligence Collection Requirements (questions or statements requesting information) and prioritized in a comprehensive, dynamic Intelligence Collection Plan. Results are monitored, and collectors are re-tasked as required.

B. (U) **Written Intelligence Products**

(U//FOUO) The FBI is authorized to conduct research, analyze information, and prepare reports and intelligence assessments (analytical products) concerning matters relevant to authorized FBI activities, such as: (i) reports and intelligence assessments (analytical product) concerning types of criminals or criminal activities; (ii) organized crime groups, terrorism, espionage, or other threats to the national security; (iii) foreign intelligence matters; or (iv) the scope and nature of criminal activity in particular geographic areas or sectors of the economy. (AGG-Dom, Part IV)

(U//FOUO) **United States Person Information:** Reports, Intelligence Assessments, and other FBI intelligence products should not contain United States person information including the names of United States corporations, if the pertinent intelligence can be conveyed without including identifying information.

(U//FOUO) FBI intelligence products, both raw and finished, serve a wide range of audiences from national-level policy and decision-makers, intelligence agencies, and state, local and tribal law enforcement agencies.

(U//FOUO) Intelligence products prepared pursuant to this Section include, but are not limited to: Domain Management, Special Events Management Threat Assessments, Intelligence Assessments, Intelligence Bulletins, Intelligence Information Reports, WMD Scientific and Technical Assessments, and Regional Field Office Assessments.

C. (U) **Intelligence Systems**

(U//FOUO) The FBI is authorized to operate intelligence, identification, tracking, and information systems in support of authorized investigative activities, or for such other or additional purposes as may be legally authorized, such as intelligence and tracking systems relating to terrorists, gangs, or organized crime groups. (AGG-Dom, Part IV)

(U//FOUO

b2
b7E

240

(U//FOUO) When developing a new database, the FBI OGC Privacy and Civil Liberties Unit must be consulted to determine if a Privacy Impact Assessment (PIA) must be prepared.

b2
b7E

D. (U)

(U//FOUO)

b2
b7E

b2
b7E

(U//FOUO)

b2
b7E

16. (U) Undisclosed Participation (UDP)

16.1. (U) Overview

(U//FOUO) Undisclosed participation (UDP) takes place when anyone acting on behalf of the FBI, including but not limited to an FBI employee or confidential human source (CHS), becomes a member or participates in the activity of an organization on behalf of the U.S. Government without disclosing FBI affiliation to an appropriate official of the organization.

A. (U) **Authorities.** The FBI derives its authority to engage in UDP in organizations as part of its investigative and intelligence collection missions from two primary sources.

(U) First, Executive Order (E.O.) 12333 broadly establishes policy for the United States Intelligence Community (USIC). Executive Order 12333 requires the adoption of procedures for undisclosed participation in organizations on behalf of elements of the USIC within the United States. Specifically, the Order provides ". . . [n]o one acting on behalf of the Intelligence Community may join or otherwise participate in any organization in the United States on behalf of the any element of the Intelligence Community without first disclosing such person's intelligence affiliation to appropriate officials of the organization, except in accordance with procedures established by the head of the Intelligence Community element concerned …. Such participation shall be authorized only if it is essential to achieving lawful purposes as determined by the Intelligence Community element head or designee." (E.O. 12333, Section 2.9, Undisclosed Participation in Organizations Within the United States). The Order also provides, at Section 2.2, that "[n]othing in [E.O. 12333] shall be construed to apply to or interfere with any authorized civil or criminal law enforcement responsibility of any department or agency."

(U) Second, in addition to its role as member of the USIC, the FBI is also the primary criminal investigative agency of the federal government with authority and responsibility to investigate all violations of federal law that are not exclusively assigned to another federal agency. This includes the investigation of crimes involving international terrorism and espionage. As a criminal investigative agency, the FBI has the authority to engage in UDP as part of a predicated investigation or an assessment.

(U//FOUO) The FBI's UDP policy is designed to incorporate the FBI's responsibilities as both a member of the USIC and as the primary criminal investigative agency of the federal government and, therefore, applies to all investigative and information collection activities of the FBI. It is intended to provide uniformity and clarity so that FBI employees have one set of standards to govern all UDP. As is the case throughout the DIOG, however, somewhat different constraints exist if the purpose of the activity is the collection of positive foreign intelligence that falls outside the FBI's law enforcement authority. Those constraints are reflected where applicable below.

B. (U//FOUO) **Mitigation of Risk.**

b2
b7E

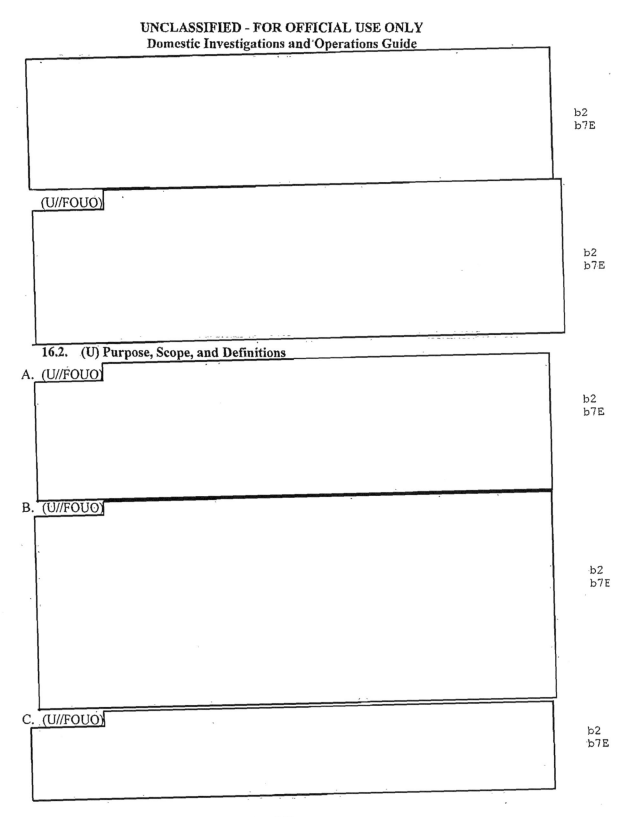

b2
b7E

(U//FOUO)

b2
b7E

16.2. (U) Purpose, Scope, and Definitions

A. (U//FOUO)

b2
b7E

B. (U//FOUO)

b2
b7E

C. (U//FOUO)

b2
b7E

1. (U//FOUO)

b2
b7E

2. (U//FOUO)

b2
b7E

3. (U//FOUO)

b2
b7E

4. (U//FOUO)

b2
b7E

D. (U//FOUO)

b2
b7E

b2
b7E

E. (U//FOUO)

b2
b7E

F. (U//FOUO)

b2
b7E

G. (U//FOUO)

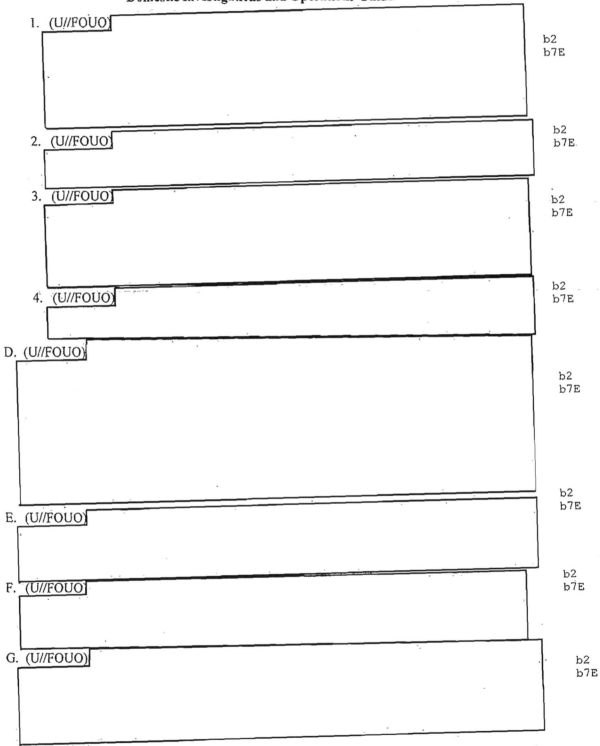

b2
b7E

b2
b7E

H. (U//FOUO)

b2
b7E

b2
1. (U//FOUO) b7E

b2
2. (U//FOUO) b7E

b2
3. (U//FOUO) b7E

b2
(U//FOUO) b7E

b2
(U//FOUO) b7E

b2
I. (U//FOUO) b7E

16.3. (U) Requirements for Approval

A. (U//FOUO)

b2
b7E

1. (U//FOUO) [redacted]   b2
b7E

2. (U//FOUO) [redacted]   b2
b7E

3. (U//FOUO) [redacted]   b2
b7E

B. (U//FOUO) Specific Requirements for General Undisclosed Participation (Non-sensitive UDP):   b2
b7E

    1. (U//FOUO) [redacted]   b2
b7E

       a. (U//FOUO) [redacted]   b2
b7E

       b. (U//FOUO) [redacted]   b2
b7E

    2. (U//FOUO) [redacted]   b2
b7E

    (U//FOUO) [redacted]

       a. (U//FOUO) [redacted]   b2
b7E

b. (U//FOUO)   b2
                                                                      b7E

c. (U//FOUO)   b2
                                                                      b5
                                                                      b7E

d. (U//FOUO)   b2.
                                                                      b5
                                                                      b7E

                                                                      b2
C. (U//FOUO)   b7E

                                                                      b2
1. (U//FOUO)   b7E

    a. (U//FOUO)   b2
                                                                      b7E

    b. (U//FOUO)   b2
                                                                      b5
                                                                      b7E

    c. (U//FOUO)   b2
                                                                      b7E

b2
b7E

b2
b7E

2. (U//FOUO)

(U//FOUO)

b2
b5
b7E

3. (U//FOUO)

b2
b7E

(U//FOUO)

b2
b7E

a. (U//FOUO)

b2
b7E

b. (U//FOUO)

b2
b5
b7E

a. (U//FOUO)

b2
b5
b7E

16.4. (U) Supervisory Approval Not Required

(U//FOUO)

b2
b7E

A. (U//FOUO)

b2
b7E

B. (U//FOUO)

b2
b7E

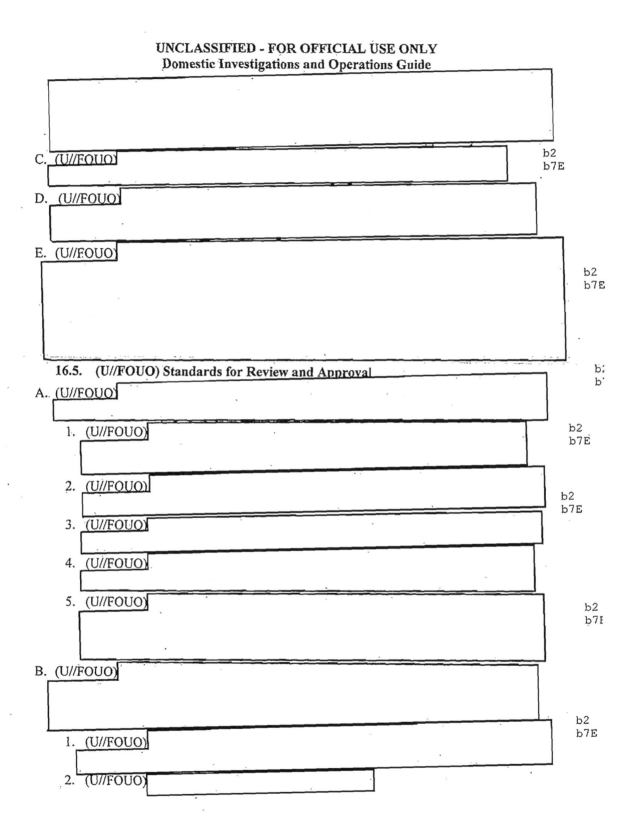

C. (U//FOUO)   b2
                                                                            b7E

D. (U//FOUO)

E. (U//FOUO)

                                                                            b2
                                                                            b7E

16.5. (U//FOUO) Standards for Review and Approval   b2
                                                                            b7
A. (U//FOUO)

    1. (U//FOUO)   b2
                                                                            b7E

    2. (U//FOUO)   b2
                                                                            b7E

    3. (U//FOUO)

    4. (U//FOUO)

    5. (U//FOUO)   b2
                                                                            b7E

B. (U//FOUO)

                                                                            b2
                                                                            b7E

    1. (U//FOUO)

    2. (U//FOUO)

C. (U//FOUO) 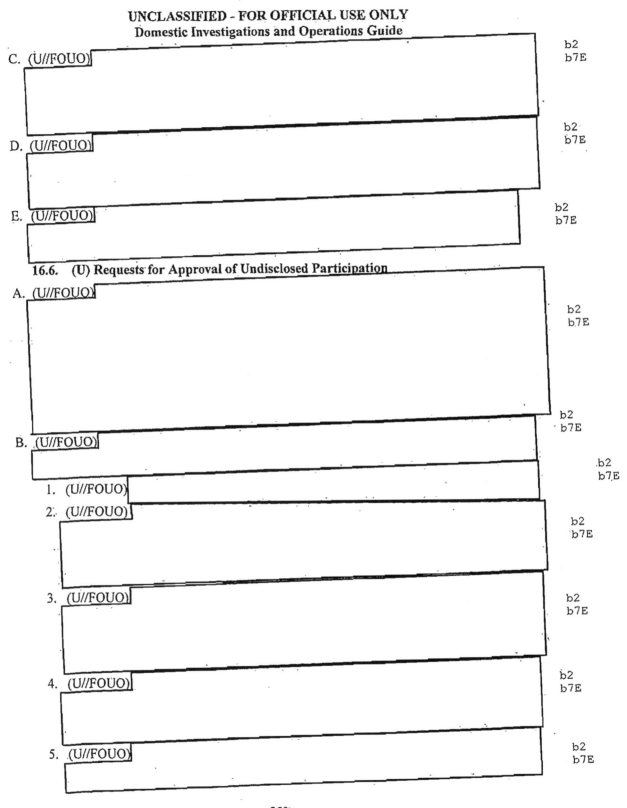   b2
b7E

D. (U//FOUO)   b2
b7E

E. (U//FOUO)   b2
b7E

16.6.   (U) Requests for Approval of Undisclosed Participation

A. (U//FOUO)   b2
b7E

    b2
b7E

B. (U//FOUO)   b2
b7E

    1. (U//FOUO)

    2. (U//FOUO)   b2
b7E

    3. (U//FOUO)   b2
b7E

    4. (U//FOUO)   b2
b7E

    5. (U//FOUO)   b2
b7E

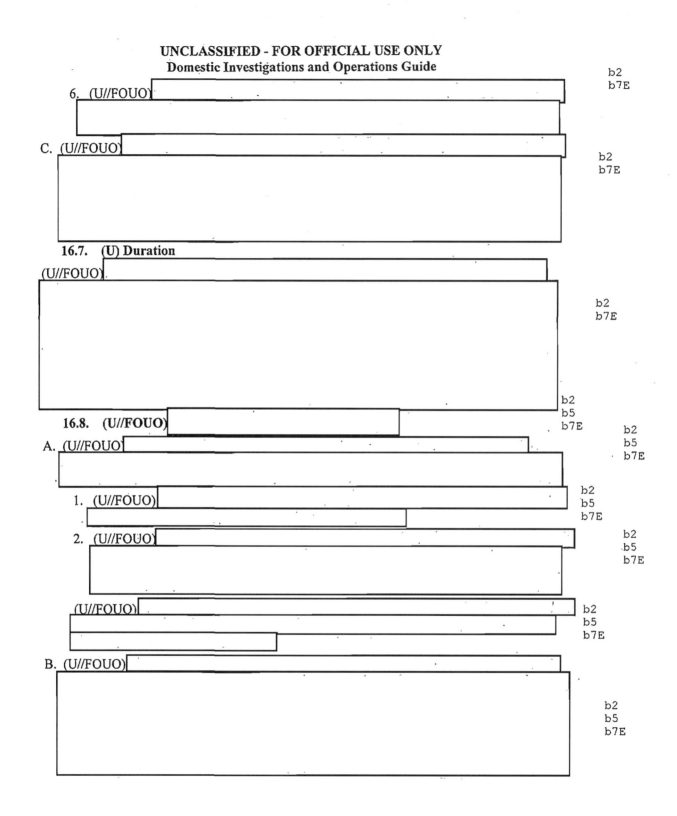

6. (U//FOUO)

C. (U//FOUO)

16.7.   (U) Duration

(U//FOUO)

16.8.   (U//FOUO)

A. (U//FOUO)

    1. (U//FOUO)

    2. (U//FOUO)

    (U//FOUO)

B. (U//FOUO)

b2
b7E

b2
b7E

b2
b7E

b2
b5
b7E

b2
b5
b7E

b2
b5
b7E

b2
b5
b7E

b2
b5
b7E

b2
b5
b7E

b2
b5
b7E

16.9. (U//FOUO) UDP EXAMPLES

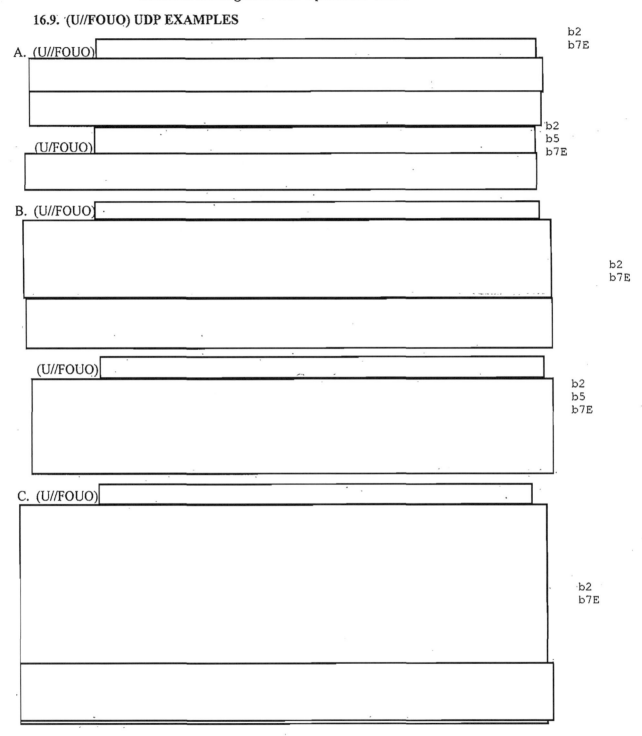

A. (U//FOUO)   b2
     b7E

(U//FOUO)   b2
     b5
     b7E

B. (U//FOUO)   b2
     b7E

(U//FOUO)   b2
     b5
     b7E

C. (U//FOUO)   b2
     b7E

(U//FOUO)

b2
b5
b7E

D. (U//FOUO)

b2
b7E

(U//FOUO)

b2
b5
b7E

E. (U//FOUO)

b2
b7E

(U//FOUO)

b2
b5
b7E

F. (U//FOUO)

b2
b7E

(U//FOUO)

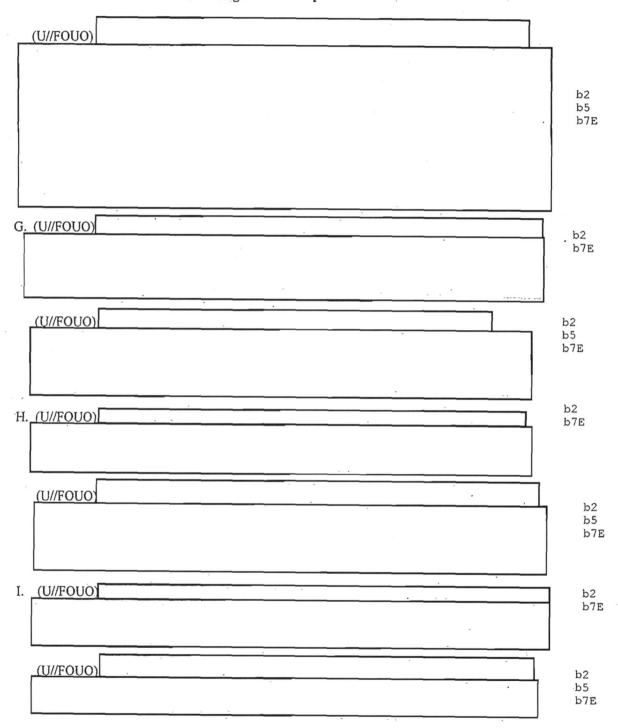

b2
b5
b7E

G. (U//FOUO)

b2
b7E

(U//FOUO)

b2
b5
b7E

H. (U//FOUO)

b2
b7E

(U//FOUO)

b2
b5
b7E

I. (U//FOUO)

b2
b7E

(U//FOUO)

b2
b5
b7E

b2
b7E

J. (U//FOUO)

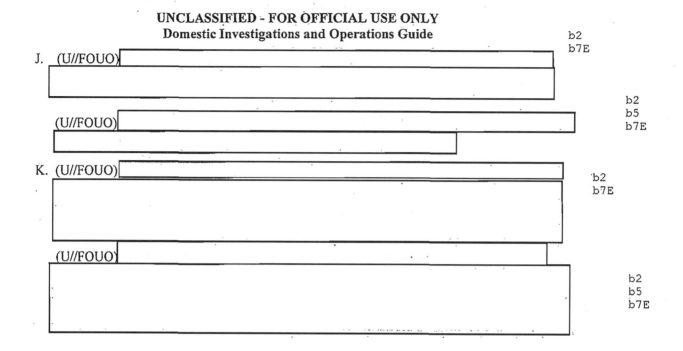

b2
b5
b7E

(U//FOUO)

K. (U//FOUO)

b2
b7E

(U//FOUO)

b2
b5
b7E

17. (U) Otherwise Illegal Activity

17.1. (U) Overview

(U//FOUO) Otherwise Illegal Activity (OIA) is conduct in the course of duties by an FBI employee (to include a UCE) or CHS which constitutes a crime under local, state, or federal law if engaged in by a person acting without authorization. Under limited circumstances, OIA can be authorized for an FBI employee or CHS to obtain information or evidence necessary for the success of an investigation under the following circumstances: (i) when that information or evidence is not reasonably available without participation in the OIA; ⎵ or (iii) when necessary to prevent serious bodily injury or death. Certain types of OIA are not authorized such as participation in an act of violence, except in self-defense, or participation in conduct that would constitute an unlawful investigative technique such an illegal wiretap.

b2
b7E

17.2. (U) Purpose and Scope

(U//FOUO) The use of OIA may be approved in the course of undercover activities or operations that involve an FBI employee or that involve use of a CHS. When approved, OIA should be limited or minimized in scope to only that which is reasonably necessary under the circumstances including the duration and geographic area to which approval applies, if appropriate.

17.3. (U//FOUO) OIA in Undercover Activity

A. (U//FOUO) **General.** The use of the undercover method is discussed in the DIOG Section 11.8. OIA is often proposed as part of an undercover scenario or in making the initial undercover contacts before the operation is approved. Specific approval for OIA must be obtained in the context of these undercover activities or operations in addition to general approval of the scenario or the operation.

B. (U//FOUO) **OIA by an FBI employee in an undercover operation relating to activity in violation of federal criminal law that does not concern a threat to the national security or foreign intelligence:** must be approved in conformity with the AGG-UCO. Approval of OIA in conformity with the AGG-UCO is sufficient and satisfies any approval requirement that would otherwise apply under the AGG-Dom. Additional discussion is provided in the Field Guide for FBI Undercover and Sensitive Operations. An SAC may approve the OIA described in subsection 17.5.

   1. (U//FOUO) When a UCE provides goods and service (reasonably unavailable to the subject except as provided by the United States government) that facilitate a felony, or its equivalent under federal, state, or local law, it is a sensitive circumstance. In these sensitive circumstances, additional authorization by an Assistant Director is required after review by the Criminal Undercover Operations Review Committee (CUORC).

   2. (U//FOUO) Participation in otherwise illegal activity that involves a significant risk of violence or physical injury requires authorization by the Director, Deputy Director, or designated Executive Assistant Director after review by the CUORC.

C. (U//FOUO) **OIA by an FBI employee in an undercover operation relating to a threat to the national security or foreign intelligence collection** must conform to the AGG-Dom.

The DOJ NSD is the approving component for OIA that requires approval beyond that authorized for SAC approval described in DIOG subsection 17.5, below. However, as authorized by the Assistant Attorney General for NSD, officials in other DOJ components may approve OIA in such investigations.

17.4. (U//FOUO) OIA for a Confidential Human Source

(U//FOUO) OIA by a CHS must be approved in conformity with the AGG-CHS and the FBI CHSPM.

17.5. (U//FOUO) Approval of OIA by a Special Agent in Charge

(U//FOUO) An SAC may authorize the following OIA for an FBI employee when consistent with other requirements of this section, the AGG-UCO, and other FBI policy:.

A. (U//FOUO) Otherwise illegal activity that would not be a felony under federal, state, local, or tribal law;

B. (U//FOUO) Consensual monitoring of communications, even if a crime under state, local, or tribal law;

(U//FOUO) **Note:** Other approvals for the consensual monitoring may apply such as that required when the consensual monitoring involves a sensitive monitoring circumstance. See DIOG Section 11.5.4.

(U//FOUO) **Note:** For those state, local and tribal governments that do not sanction or provide a law enforcement exception available to the FBI for one-party consent recording of communications with persons within their jurisdiction, the SAC must approve the consensual monitoring of communications as an OIA. Prior to the SAC authorizing the OIA, one-party consent must be acquired. The SAC may delegate the OIA approval authority to an ASAC or SSA.

C. (U//FOUO) The controlled purchase, receipt, delivery, or sale of drugs, stolen property, or other contraband;

D. (U//FOUO) The payment of bribes;

(U//FOUO) **Note:** the payment of bribes and the amount of such bribes in a public corruption matter may be limited by other FBI policy; see the CID PG.

E. (U//FOUO) The making of false representations in concealment of personal identity or the true ownership of a proprietary; and

F. (U//FOUO) Conducting a money laundering transaction or transactions involving an aggregate amount not exceeding $1 million.

(U//FOUO) **Exception:** An SAC may not authorize an activity that may constitute material support to terrorism, a violation of export control laws, or a violation of laws that concern proliferation of weapons of mass destruction. In such an investigation, an SAC may authorize an activity that may otherwise violate prohibitions of material support to terrorism only according to standards established by the Director of the FBI and agreed to by the Assistant Attorney General for National Security. (AGG-Dom, Part V.C.3)

17.6. (U//FOUO) Standards for Review and Approval of OIA

(U//FOUO) No official may recommend or approve participation by an FBI employee in OIA unless the participation is justified:

A. (U//FOUO) To obtain information or evidence necessary for the success of the investigation and not reasonably available without participation in the otherwise illegal activity;

B. (U//FOUO) [   ] or   b2
                                                                   b7E

C. (U//FOUO) To prevent death or serious bodily injury.

17.7. (U//FOUO) OIA not authorized

(U//FOUO) The following activities may not be authorized for an FBI employee:

A. (U//FOUO) Directing or participating in acts of violence;

> (U//FOUO) **Note:** Self-defense and defense of others. FBI employees are authorized to engage in any lawful use of force, including the use of force in self-defense or defense of others in the lawful discharge of their duties.

B. (U//FOUO) Activities whose authorization is prohibited by law, including unlawful investigative methods, such as illegal, non-consensual, electronic surveillance or illegal searches.

> (U//FOUO) **Note:** Subparagraph B includes activities that would violate protected constitutional or federal statutory rights in the absence of a court order or warrant such as illegal wiretaps and searches.

17.8. (U//FOUO) Emergency Situations

(U//FOUO) Without prior approval, an FBI employee may engage in OIA that could be authorized under this section only if necessary to meet an immediate threat to the safety of persons or property or to the national security, or to prevent the compromise of an investigation or the loss of a significant investigative opportunity. In such a case, prior to engaging in the OIA, every effort should be made by the FBI employee to consult with the SAC, and by the SAC to consult with the USAO or appropriate DOJ Division where the authorization of that office or Division would be required unless the circumstances preclude such consultation. Cases in which OIA occur pursuant to this paragraph without the authorization required must be reported as soon as possible to the SAC, and by the SAC to FBIHQ and to the USAO or appropriate DOJ Division.